COURAGE *for* CAREGIVERS
SUSTENANCE FOR THE JOURNEY
IN COMPANY WITH
HENRI J. M. NOUWEN

THE STORY OF CAREGIVING SERIES

MARJORIE J. THOMPSON

Church Health | Henri Nouwen Society
MEMPHIS, TN | TORONTO, ONTARIO

Courage for Caregivers: Sustenance for the Journey in Company with Henri J. M. Nouwen

© 2017 The Henri Nouwen Legacy Trust and Church Health Center of Memphis, Inc.

Created by the Henri Nouwen Legacy Trust and Church Health Center of Memphis, Inc.

Written by Marjorie J. Thompson

Edited by Susan Martins Miller

Stephen Lazarus, editorial advisor, Henri Nouwen Society

Designed by Lizy Heard

Material written by Henri Nouwen
© Henri Nouwen Legacy Trust 2017

ISBN: 9781621440598

Printed in the United States of America.

COVER AND INTERIOR ARTWORK BY MATTHEW CHAPMAN

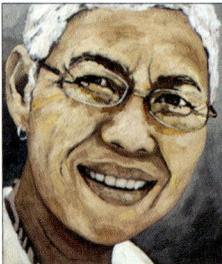

"I believe that our deepest desire is to connect meaningfully with others. For me, portraiture is a way of exploring the human story, as stories are told in the lines of our faces."
—Matt Chapman
PORTRAIT ARTIST | TORONTO, CANADA

Table of Contents

Acknowledgments

AS ONE WHO KNEW Henri Nouwen personally, and whose life and ministry has been shaped in countless ways by his presence and teaching, I consider it a high privilege to have been asked to write *Courage for Caregivers*. It has given me a priceless opportunity to revisit my years of elder care alongside my husband, John Mogabgab, who worked with Henri for five years at Yale Divinity School. More, it has afforded me the great joy of renewing my acquaintance with Henri's wonderfully generous gifts of written and spoken material—a true treasury of spiritual wisdom.

I am much indebted to all who have helped in the visioning, development, and production of this book with its related resources. Karen Pascal, executive director of the Henri Nouwen Society, invited me to take on the writing task and offered encouraging support all along the way. The consultation Karen called together in September of 2016 helped shape a vision of caregiving with the distinctive imprint of Henri's wisdom on care. My deep gratitude to those in attendance, including Sue Mosteller, Stephen Lazarus, Rachel Davis, Judith Leckie, Angela Caffrey, and Judith Cooke, several of whom offered continued support by reading and critiquing early chapter drafts. Special thanks to Stephen Lazarus, editorial advisor for the Henri Nouwen Society, who sent an array of quotes suited to the caregiving theme and supplied many needed citations, helping me to negotiate Henri's voluminous writings.

From the side of our Church Health partners, I owe much to Rachel Davis, who initiated me into the mysteries of audio-recording cell phone interviews and served as liaison with Church Health principles involved in supporting the project. Church Health founder and CEO Dr. Scott Morris has championed the collaborative project, and Brad Martin, longtime friend to Church Health and board member, has generously underwritten the endeavor. Finally, I could not have accomplished this writing without the thoughtful and experienced eye of Susan Martins Miller, whose constructive critique and fine-tuned sensibilities made her the ideal editor, and who contributed directly to the writing of Appendix B, which has widened the ways this book can be used even as awareness of caregiving needs expands.

Not least, I wish to express my heartfelt gratitude for those who gave me permission to conduct and tape interviews. They gave hours of precious time to share their own remarkable stories of giving or receiving care, along with inspiring spiritual and practical insights to share with our readers. Thanks, and a deep bow, to Lindsey Yeskoo, Donna Thomson, Karen Shepherd, Vanessa Beasley, Cyndy Wacker, Judy Hazlett, Tracy Hilts, and Michelle O'Rourke.

Preface

I TOOK A RATHER circuitous route on the way to discovering Henri Nouwen.

During my time as a television producer in the 80s and 90s, I produced five seasons of a current affairs program—topical events viewed and discussed from a Judeo-Christian perspective. The series featured interesting and varied guests on each episode. Newsmakers, authors, artists, business people, environmentalists, activists, politicians, and pundits were a grand menagerie of engaging and articulate individuals.

As much from personal curiosity as from professional inquiry, I quickly acquired the habit of asking each guest what she or he was currently reading. I wanted to know what fueled them, what fired their passions, their minds, their spirits.

I anticipated that the reading selections they offered would be as eclectic as the group itself. However, to my surprise, books by a spiritual writer named Henri Nouwen were mentioned and recommended again and again, titles such as *The Return of the Prodigal Son*, *The Wounded Healer*, *Gracias!* and *Life of the Beloved*.

I don't recall exactly which of Henri's books I read first, but I do remember the feeling I had when I began reading. It was as if the author was writing about *me*, as if he was looking into my heart, parsing and describing *my* life's experience. My hopes, my hurts, my brokenness. I was consoled. I was inspired. I was hooked.

A few years after being introduced to his books, I tracked Henri down at his home at L'Arche Daybreak, situated just north of Toronto. And when I say I tracked Henri down, that's exactly what I mean. Henri was an extremely busy man. Besides contributing to the care of core members at L'Arche, Henri was also the community's spiritual director. In addition, he traveled extensively. The popularity of his books made him a much sought-after speaker in North America and beyond. Yet he still made time to write, to pray, and to respond to the many letters he received each day from friends, colleagues, and even complete strangers asking him for counseling and spiritual encouragement.

He reluctantly—yet graciously—agreed to allow me to feature him in one of my programs. Less than two years later, Henri died of a heart attack on his way to do a documentary in Russia on *The Return of the Prodigal Son*. Like everyone who knew him, either personally or through his books, I was shocked and heartbroken, but I knew instinctively that Henri's legacy would live on. Henri himself had written that if our deepest human desire is to give ourselves to others, then death will be a final gift that will continue to bear fruit long after we die.

Henri died, but he never died. His legacy lives on and continues to bear fruit in the lives of many people who, like me, stumble upon his books in any number of ways.

Henri recognized that God's love is not diminished by our trials, losses, and brokenness; rather it's in the midst of our pain where we often experience it most deeply. In your role as a caregiver, whether in a professional capacity or one who was thrust into the role by circumstance, I pray that you will find comfort, encouragement, and *courage* within these pages. And may you continue to find the depth of God's love in your life as Henri found in his.

Karen Pascal,
Executive Director
Henri Nouwen Society
Toronto, Ontario

Foreword

I FIRST MET HENRI NOUWEN when I was a student at Yale Divinity School and he was on the faculty. He was coming into his popularity as a spiritual writer at the time, and as a result he had groupies on campus who hung on every word he said and seemed to follow him everywhere he went. It wasn't long before I joined those who were drawn into wanting to be closer to him. He was a magician with words, and in five minutes he made you think he had used a straw and could directly access the marrow of God. In the fall of 1978, I was with him in the hallway outside the mail room. I told him I needed help to better find a sense of peace in my life that would let me listen to God speaking to me and my sense of calling around the issues of faith and health for the poor.

He said, "Over the Christmas break you should go spend a week in silence at Taizé."

"That sounds great. I'll do it." I then asked him, "Where is Taizé?"

He looked at me the way I would if someone said, "Where is Yankee stadium?"

"In southern France," he replied.

Of course it is, I thought. And so, I began to make plans to go. God was waiting for me there.

I did go to Taizé, where I talked to the cows and confirmed my suspicion that the cloth I was cut from was woven more for action than contemplation. During my week of silence, nothing of long-standing, profound significance happened. And yet, for the last 40 years, a week rarely goes by that I don't think of being there.

When I returned to Yale, I began going almost every evening to Compline services led by Henri Nouwen at five in the afternoon. Beneath the main chapel at Yale Divinity School is a smaller chapel that Henri had made his own. Every day a small group, no more than a dozen, would gather for a 20-minute service. Henri gave a brief homily, said a few prayers, and then offered communion. I loved going, mostly because of his charisma and my feeling that he knew something about connecting to God I needed to know. He focused on prayer and contemplation but believed in social justice. He had long hands with a broad span from thumb to little finger, and he spoke every sentence using his hands. I couldn't take my eyes off him. The rest of my time at Yale, I tried to learn as much as I could from Henri. I never stopped loving to hear him preach and teach. Years later, when I was in my medical training and had the opportunity to hear him speak in the city where I then lived, I wasn't sure he would remember me, but he reached out with those huge hands and pulled me close to him. We talked about my going to medical school and my plans for the future. He made me proud of what I was doing.

Now more than two decades after his death, I have felt his embrace once again when the Henri Nouwen Society and Legacy Trust became interested in the work of Church Health, the organization I founded in 1987 and which still cares for the medical needs of people in low-wage jobs. In addition, Church Health publishes resources around themes of faith and health. It's been our privilege to partner with the Henri Nouwen Society and Legacy Trust first on *Hope for Caregivers: A 42-Day Devotional in Company with Henri J. M. Nouwen* and now on *Courage for Caregivers: Sustenance for the Journey in Company with Henri J. M. Nouwen.*

That I could have a part in bringing to fruition resources around a subject so central to Henri's life and teaching brings me great personal joy. In addition, what mattered so deeply to Henri richly reflects an issue important to the mission of Church Health in our effort to speak to an ever-growing need among individuals and faith communities.

As Henri's words continue to remind us, each of us is God's beloved. I can think of no theme more significant to carry forward into the courageous ministry of giving and receiving care.

Rev. Scott Morris, MD
Founder and CEO
Church Health
Memphis, Tennessee

Beginnings

HENRI NOUWEN, OUR SPIRITUAL COMPANION

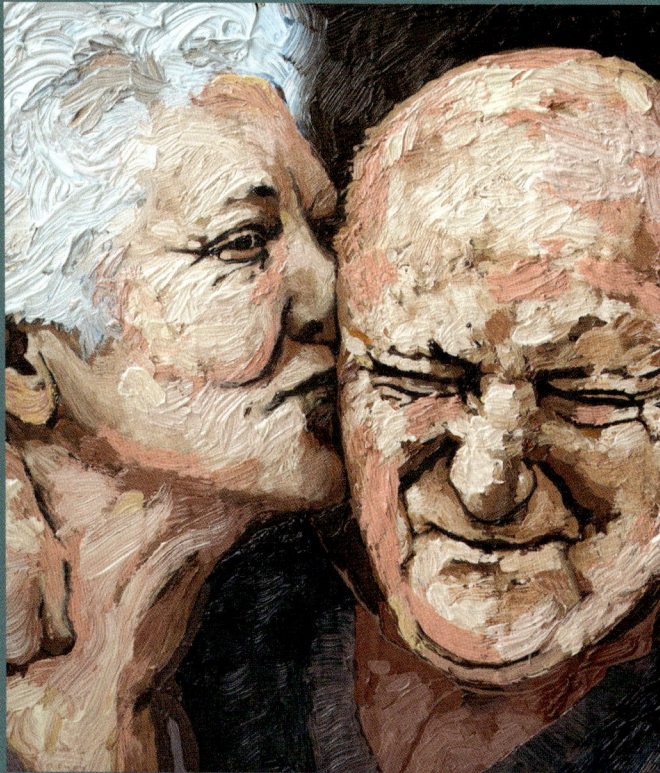

THIS BOOK IS written to provide a rich spiritual perspective on the experience of giving and receiving care. The views offered here are deeply rooted in Christian tradition—broadly framed to welcome people of many denominations, as well as those who may be unaffiliated yet are seeking a transcendent compass in life.

Henri Nouwen—beloved spiritual writer, teacher, and pastor—will be our spiritual companion and primary spiritual guide as we wrestle with the challenges and identify the joys of caregiving. Henri had much to say on the subject of care across the arc of his ministry. A Dutch Catholic priest who reached across denominational boundaries, he touched the hearts of people worldwide. His humility and vulnerability revealed our shared humanity. Deeply conscious of his own weakness, limitation, and longing, he gave powerful witness to the grace of God's infinitely tender love for all. Henri was not afraid to acknowledge the "dark night" of our human journeys, nor was he shy to proclaim the great hope and joy of our faith.

Above all, Henri delighted to share his experience of God's love, hoping that it not only might illumine his most deeply felt and hard-won spiritual truth but also open wider doors into our own experience of the same grace. As he put it, "My hope is that the description of God's love in my life will give you the freedom and courage to discover—and maybe also describe—God's love in yours.[1]

Henri was a natural spiritual companion to everyone he befriended on his life's journey. Countless people found him a trustworthy guide through struggles and triumphs. May his simple words and deep wisdom help to sustain us as well.

OUR STORIED LIVES

Stories are essential to our understanding of human life. They help us make sense of the narrative of our own lives. Great teachers have always used stories to illustrate and illuminate important truths. Jesus was a consummate storyteller, capable of conjuring up a parable on the spot to bring a spiritual truth to life in the hearts of his hearers. Most of us are familiar with Jesus' greatest parables, like the Good Samaritan and the Prodigal Son. All of his parables pointed his hearers to deep truths about God's character and kingdom. The most powerful human stories keep working in our hearts over time. Some become beacons of light for a lifetime.

Our personal stories may not seem so elevated, but they are equally significant for our self-understanding and can become light for others as well. To tell a story requires some measure of reflection. We take the raw experience of life and digest it in memory, thought, and feeling. We piece together the sequence of events, our felt experience, and the recollections of others who were part of the situation. As we do this, a frame of meaning often emerges that gives the story cohesion. Sometimes we carry the meaning in a narrative—a word picture of unfolding events, characters involved, and fragments of dialogue. Sometimes we express the meaning in terms of insight, wisdom, depth of emotion, or spiritual growth. A sense of higher purpose in the stories of our lives can come through reflection on our experience over time. Also, the lens of another person's story may help us to see a larger picture in our circumstances. Our stories communicate who we are, how we mature, and how we connect.

In these pages, we are privileged to draw on several stories shared by caregivers and care receivers in various situations. These individuals share perspectives on both the challenges and gifts of their care experience. They also share words of encouragement with those of us who—in the trenches of daily care—struggle with an abundance of complexity and uncertainty.

Appendix C features condensed versions of these stories, while the main chapters incorporate elements of several for illustration.

Such stories keep us grounded in the situations of real people like us, give us broader perspective on the experience of caregiving, and help us find new ways to see and tell our own stories. Along with Henri's wisdom, the voices of these caregivers and care receivers will enrich our experience and understanding.

CAREGIVING: UNIVERSAL AND UNIQUE

The seemingly endless routines and responsibilities of caregiving can make us feel profoundly isolated. Indeed, many of us are physically alone for long stretches in our care of another person. Yet in a larger sense, we are by no means alone. Caring is a universal experience in human life. Our friend Henri would say that to be human is to care! This truth undergirded Henri's life and teaching. In one instance he writes, "To care is the most human of all gestures,"[2] and in another, "caring is the privilege of every person and is at the heart of being human."[3] We are very much together in the remarkable adventure of faithful caregiving.

It is virtually certain that, within our life span, most of us will have the opportunity to take on primary responsibility for the care of at least one other human being. While this may feel sobering or daunting, caregiving is also one of the most meaningful tasks we could ever give ourselves to. For some, the opportunities will abound. In today's world, it is not uncommon for a person to know the joys and rigors of raising children, caring for a spouse with serious illness, and juggling the demands of care for aging parents—usually, but not always, spread out over several decades. When caregiving responsibilities for different generations overlap in time, the challenges are greatly compounded.

Most of us know the joys and heartaches of caring for growing children. We are well aware how much time, attention, and energy are required to parent well, particularly when our kids are most vulnerable and dependent. Children with typically developing abilities pose ample challenges to their caregivers as they grow. In the process, parents know exhaustion, frustration, satisfaction, and exhilaration by turns. On the whole, however, the physical demands of parenting decrease as these children mature and become increasingly capable of handling needs on their own.

It is quite a different story when children are born with or develop serious physical or intellectual disabilities. Parents who must give their medically fragile children rigorous care, attention, and emotional support—day and night—carry immense levels of stress. If their child's condition is chronic and incurable, such stresses do not diminish with time. These are some of the most challenging of all caregiving circumstances, echoed in varying degrees at the other end of the life spectrum by care for the fragile elderly. Yet such challenges can strike at any age. Consider: the couple unexpectedly caring for a young adult son after he suffered an accident that left him a paraplegic with a fully alert mind; the sibling who copes with a brother or sister battling depression and addiction; the middle-aged spouse immersed in care for a life partner suffering from sudden stroke, inoperable cancer, or a degenerative disease.

Along with varieties of circumstance, settings for care can differ widely. Many of us engage in caregiving primarily within our personal homes or nearby family homes. For others, the primary setting will be care facilities such as hospitals, rehabilitation centers, assisted care facilities, specialized group homes, residential hospices, or nursing homes. Settings may alternate between private homes and professional care centers as medical or family circumstances change. In our geographically far-flung families today, caring for elders is frequently managed at a distance, with adult children making repeated trips to assist aging parents in another state. Every setting comes with its own advantages and disadvantages.

We as caregivers are also diverse: family members, friends, persons employed as aides for in-home care, health care professionals, and pastoral care ministers. Care professionals may have personal caregiving responsibilities to manage alongside their day jobs, placing them in near-constant care roles. In this, they share the realities so familiar to those immersed in the demands of unceasing care for high-needs family members.

Courage for Caregivers is primarily directed toward ordinary people of faith engaged in giving care to family members at home or in nearby settings. Yet given the complexities of modern health care, the natural connections of our lives, and our great need for support amid the demands of caregiving, we trust that what is offered here will also be useful to care professionals, care ministry teams, and family or friends who simply wish to understand and support caregivers they love who are laboring "in the trenches." We are, after all, in this human predicament together!

The Mutuality of Caregiving

SHARED SUFFERING AND COMPASSION

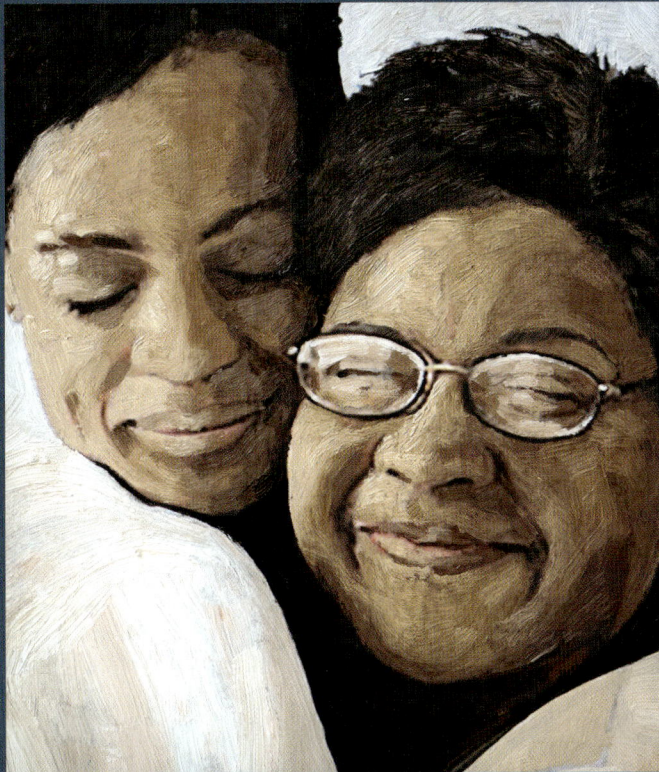

H ENRI BROUGHT PARTICULAR insights to our experience of caring for each other. We can identify three keys to explore:

1. *Care is not cure*: true care allows us to be comfortable with weakness.
2. *Care expresses and expands our compassion*, understood as suffering with others.
3. *Care draws us into profound mutuality*, both in shared vulnerability and shared gifts.

HENRI'S WISDOM ON CARE VERSUS CURE

A helpful starting point is Henri's insistence that "care is distinctly different from cure."[1] Henri believed that our care for the elderly helps to reveal this truth with singular clarity, because more than other age groups "the elderly confront us all with the fact that the concept of a final cure is an illusion."[2] In a culture fixated on problem solving, we are often more interested in cure than care. Care professionals like doctors, psychologists, and social workers are trained to evaluate their competence by standard measures of successful treatment. Yet, Henri notes, "our altruistic intention to cure the ills of others has oriented us toward success in the eyes of others."[3] Success tends to build a sense of power and prestige in those who can cure. While we are surely happy for effective treatment, the drive to cure may not always result in true care. "Many people have returned from a clinic cured but depersonalized" by aloof or arrogant professionals. It is a real but often unconscious temptation for care professionals to relate to their patients "as the powerful to the powerless, the knower to the ignorant."[4]

In contrast to cure, Henri lifts up the beauty and value of authentic care:

What is care? The word finds its origin in the word *kara*, which means to lament, to mourn, to participate in suffering, to share in pain. To care is to cry out with those who are ill, confused, lonely, isolated, and forgotten, and to recognize their pains in our own heart. To care is to enter into the world of those who are broken and powerless and to establish there a fellowship of the weak. To care is to be present to those who suffer, and to stay present, even when nothing can be done to change their situation.[5]

Care is the context within which cure, where possible, may be received as gift. Yet, Henri assures us, when we cannot cure we can still care. It is always possible to say—through our presence, listening, words, or gestures—"I see your pain. I cannot take it away, but I won't leave you alone."[6]

> *For too long care has been conceived of as either practitioner-centered or patient-centered. In actuality, the healing relationship has always been a crucible for mutual transformation.*
> —SAKI SANTORELLI

SUFFERING AND COMPASSION

Henri helps us to embrace care for others as a way of participating in their suffering. Those of us with long experience in caregiving for family members will know two sides to this suffering: the difficulty, weakness, and pain of those who receive our care; and our struggle as caregivers to balance family expectations, work responsibilities, time constraints, limited energy, and perhaps sporadic efforts at self-care. There are seasons when we feel we are barely staying afloat on a sea of swirling changes and swelling demands.

Since suffering is a reality on both sides of the care relationship, one constructive thing we can do is to ask ourselves long-term questions like these:

- How do I choose to face pain or distress with courage, hope, even curiosity?
- How might I not only endure but embrace these circumstances?
- What can I learn, here and now, that serves my growth in love?

As we engage our suffering and the suffering of others with courage, we discover growing compassion. Henri's friend Parker Palmer likes to say that there are two ways a heart can break: It can be shattered into a thousand shards that explode and implode to wound others and oneself; or it can *break open* to receive more reality, insight, and love. A heart that breaks open under the pressure of suffering becomes more compassionate. Henri once wrote, "My true call is to look the suffering Jesus in the eyes and not be crushed by his pain, but to receive it in my heart and let it bear the fruit of compassion."[7]

The term *compassion* is rooted in the Latin *pati* (to bear or suffer) and *cum* (with). Compassion means "to bear with" or "suffer with." It is closely connected with empathy which shares the Latin root *pati*, and signifies an ability to feel with the other. Yet while there is a strong impulse in our heart to feel with others, there is an equally powerful resistance to feeling too much! As Henri points out,

> Compassion is hard because it requires the inner disposition to go with others to the place where they are weak, vulnerable ... and broken. But this is not our spontaneous response to suffering. What we desire most is to do away with suffering by fleeing from it or finding a quick cure for it.[8]

How many are the ways we recoil from physical and mental anguish! Suffering is a universal human experience from which no one escapes in this world. Yet no human experience raises so many profound and painful questions about the meaning and purpose of our earthly lives. Although we may ask such questions of people we hope are wiser than we, the real audience for our deepest questions is always God. Anguished questioning of God in relation to suffering is age-old, and never fully resolved by reason.

When we suffer greatly, painful questions fly from our hearts like flaming arrows: Why is this happening? What have I done to deserve this? Is God angry with me? Why doesn't God heal me? Will God ever answer my prayers? We ask similar questions on behalf of those we love, especially when their suffering is hard to bear.

> *The question, "Why?" spontaneously emerges.*
> *"Why me?" "Why now?" "Why here?" It is so arduous*
> *to live without an answer to this "Why?"*
> —HENRI NOUWEN

Behind our questions lie the eruption of difficult feelings: physical, mental, and emotional hurt; a deep sense of unfairness and consequent anger; sorrow and grief over loss; numbness and incomprehension; fear and uncertainty; helplessness and despair. Henri was deeply acquainted with these hard feelings. By example he encouraged us to be honest and realistic about them. As we explore the challenges of caregiving, we will look at stories that help us acknowledge and name our strong feelings of pain, fear, frustration, and exhaustion.

Yet Henri also keenly understood how faith sustains and strengthens us in our suffering. He assures us that before it is anything else, the mystery of salvation is this: God came to us in Jesus not to take our pains away but to share them with us. Through his passion he cried out alongside us in our agonies, our incomprehension, our loneliness and felt abandonment. He entered so fully into the human experience, and drank so deeply the bitter cup of our misery, that nothing of human suffering is now alien to God. All our suffering is held in God's heart and embraced by divine love.

There can be no human beings who are completely alone in their sufferings since God, in and through Jesus, has become Emmanuel, God with us. It belongs to the center of our faith that God is a faithful God, a God who did not want us to ever be alone, but who wanted to understand—and stand under—all that is human. The Good News of the Gospel, therefore, is not that God wanted to take our suffering away, but that God became part of it.
—HENRI NOUWEN

Jesus comes into human life revealing God's humility (Philippians 2:5–8). In Jesus, God stoops to become small and weak with us in a manger birth. In Jesus, God welcomes the neglected, the feared, the despised, and the broken in a mission of compassionate transformation. In Jesus, God takes on our suffering and death in complete solidarity. Beyond his earthly life, Jesus invites us to share symbolically in his suffering every time we "eat this bread and drink this cup," remembering his death and resurrection. Henri speaks of this cup:

> Jesus' cup is the cup of sorrow, not just his own sorrow but the sorrow of the whole human race. It is a cup full of physical, mental, and spiritual anguish. ... It is the cup

full of bitterness. Who wants to drink it? ... Too much pain to hold, too much suffering to embrace, too much agony to live through. Why, then, could he still say yes? ... beyond all the abandonment experienced in body and mind Jesus still had a spiritual bond with the one he called Abba. He possessed a trust beyond betrayal, a surrender beyond despair, a love beyond all fears.[9]

Jesus never promises that we will escape our own suffering, but rather invites us to take up our cross and follow him. He asks if we can drink the cup he drinks, knowing we can only do so the same way he did—as "a deep spiritual yes to Abba, the lover of his wounded heart."[10] He assures us that he will be with us in our struggle to say yes—with us to the end of the age (Matthew 28:20), and even beyond what we perceive as the end of life: "I go to prepare a place for you. And ... I will come again and take you to myself" (John 14:2–3). Jesus' suffering was not the final word, and neither is ours. "Was it not necessary that the Messiah should suffer these things and then enter into his glory?" (Luke 24:26). The apostle Paul assures us that as we die with Christ, so we shall enter into his resurrected life. These are all powerful promises to hold—and allow to hold us—when we are grieved by the sufferings of those we care for, and worn down by the relentlessness of giving care.

CARE AND THE TREASURE OF MUTUALITY

While care involves us unavoidably in suffering, it would be a great mistake to imagine that sharing pain is the most central feature of faithful care! Yes, pain is a realistic part of care, but so too are profound blessings and unexpected joys. Henri expresses joyful aspects of caregiving as he describes the deep mutuality that shapes these relationships: "In the very act of caring for another, you and I possess a great treasure. ... Caregiving carries within it an opportunity for inner healing, liberation, and transformation for the one being cared for and for the one who cares."[11]

Henri illustrates this mutuality with a story of his experience at the L'Arche Community of Daybreak, where he lived in a community setting with individuals living with disabilities and cared for Adam—a severely disabled young man who could not walk, speak, or care for his needs in any way. At first Henri assumed that he could not develop a relationship with someone who couldn't speak. What he discovered over time was that Adam had his own ways of communicating, and was capable of offering a very real and profound presence. Henri writes,

> Eventually I found myself confiding my secrets to him, ... telling him about my frustrations, ... and my prayer life. What was so amazing ... was the gradual realization that Adam was really there for me, listening with his whole being and offering me a safe place to be. ... Adam was becoming my teacher, taking me by the hand, walking with me in my confusion through the wilderness of my life.[12]

In caring for Adam, Henri began to recognize his own inner handicaps, less visible but just as real as Adam's physical and mental disabilities. In the peaceful, steady presence of Adam, "I was faced with a very insecure, needy, and fragile person: myself." Henri realized then that he saw Adam as the strong one.[13]

Many who have cared for people with serious illness or disability know a similar experience. Christopher deVinck wrote a book about his brother, Oliver, who from birth could not see, walk, or talk. DeVinck shows how Oliver was responsible for action, courage, love and insight in his family. This was a household where tragedy was transformed into joy![14]

Henri helps us to see our shared human vulnerability as a source of belonging, comfort, and community. We are "wounded healers" for each other.[15] By acknowledging our own wounds, we can bring an authentic healing presence to others in pain. In our common weakness we more easily recognize one another as beloved children of the same God, whose forgiving grace holds us in a unity far deeper than our superficial differences. "Those who ask for care invite us to listen to our own pains, to know our own wounds, and to face our own brokenness."[16] Thus, "one of the most beautiful characteristics of the compassionate life is that there is always a mutuality of giving and receiving. Anyone who has truly entered into the compassionate life ... will express deep gratitude for the gifts received from those they came to help. Joy is the secret gift of compassion."[17]

> *The cup of sorrow, inconceivable as it seems, is also the cup of joy. Only when we discover this in our own life can we consider drinking it.*
> —HENRI NOUWEN

In caring for each other, we slowly enter into the wisdom that suffering and joy are inseparable. Paradoxically, each creates the condition for the other side of reality to be experienced more deeply. Our next two chapters will offer stories to help us explore each side of this paradox.

The Challenges of Caregiving
NAMING AND EMBRACING

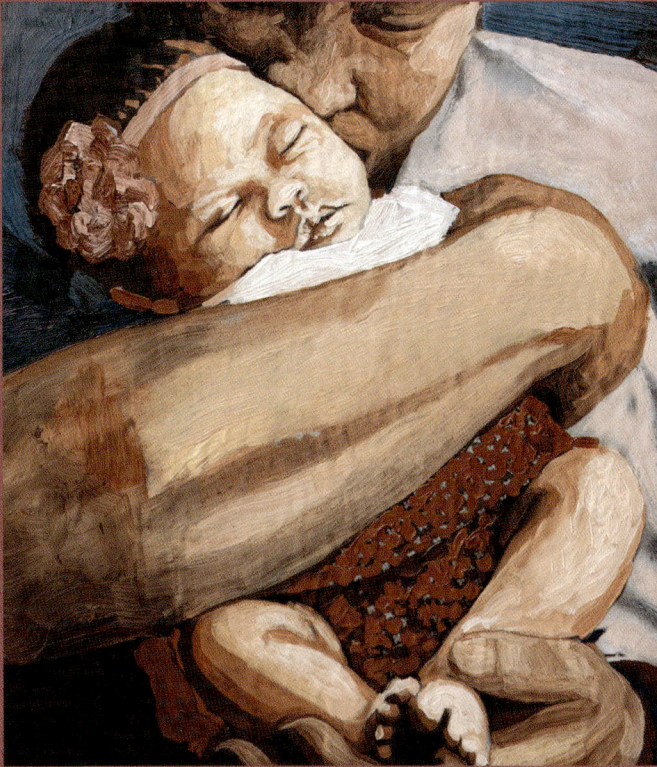

W E HAVE IDENTIFIED THE paradoxical truth that suffering and joy are mysteriously intertwined. It is time to face directly into the hard side of this paradox—the many challenges of giving and receiving care. As Henri lifts up the mutuality of caregiving, he clearly sees challenges on both sides of the relationship: "Many of us know from experience how hard it is to simply be a caregiver. At the same time, we may need to be reminded of how hard it is to be cared for. It isn't easy either way!"[1] Anyone involved with intense or long-term care knows just how difficult and complex it can be. We will look at these challenges first from the perspective of caregivers, then through the eyes of those receiving care.

I draw on several caregiver stories, among which my own will feature prominently as the one I know best. They are offered to help evoke the issues we want to reflect on in our own circumstances. Through imagination, the stories of others can join a conversation with ours. Deeply important to these conversations are the spiritual insights and perspectives we discover. They encourage us to see the richness of our lived experience and give us ways to engage in life-sustaining spiritual practice. Henri's wisdom will continue to thread in and out of the fabric we are weaving through these conversations.

CHALLENGES FOR THE CAREGIVER

Starting in 2002, my husband, John, and I cared for our mothers in a newly built home. For 20 months, we had both my mother (Jean) and my mother-in-law (Winifred, nicknamed Bab). Bab was with us for eleven years and died just shy of her hundredth birthday. Many challenges—illness, disability, anxiety, fatigue, and grief—shaped our lives for an extended stretch of time. As Henri observed, caring is an act of participating in the common suffering that is the lot of human life.

MY STORY WITH JEAN

My mother's needs were primarily physical. Her mind was blessedly sharp, her senses acute, her inward life grounded in faith and spiritual vision. Jean was neither sentimental nor afraid of dying. But with advanced chronic obstructive pulmonary disorder (COPD, in late symptoms indistinguishable from emphysema), she had very little energy. Four years before her death she suffered a heart attack. Increasingly her breath was restricted by both lung disease and heart failure.

Jean needed a great deal of help physically and was highly susceptible to chest infections, each one threatening her end. Our home was filled with oxygen equipment—a constantly sighing compressor, yards of tubing upstairs and down, a tall back-up tank in case of electrical outages. Uncertainty dominated our lives. Jean did not expect to live long. Over the course of 20 months her condition lurched up and down like a dingy on raging seas, with no steady horizon in sight. Even with paid caregivers for several hours each weekday, evening and weekend care fell mostly to me—alongside full-time work and an hour-and-a half daily commute. John helped as he could, but Jean was my mother and looked largely to me for help with her physical care needs. Through the last six months of her life under home hospice care, I truly felt like I was "hanging on by my fingernails."

During this time I faced a number of challenges. Of these, the most interesting was taking responsibility for Jean's care in ways that respected her limited autonomy and gave her meaningful choices within the parameters of our home life. Part of this dynamic was a delicate balance between needing to be parental in some respects—reversing the traditional roles—yet always remembering that she remained my mother. Jean knew the entire span of my life in a way I could never know the fullness of hers—and her memory was good! Because her mind was sound, the authority of decision-making in relation to medical care and financial choices remained in her hands with supportive help from her adult children. Yet I eventually took the liberty to sort her mail and discard sensationalist flyers for financial "bonanzas" and herbal cure-alls that arrived daily. Like many elderly people in poor health she was susceptible to the claims made by mail scams, no matter how I tried to dissuade her. When I saw that they drained not only her limited energy but her meager checkbook, I took a "parental prerogative" to protect her from her own vulnerabilities in this regard.

Of course, from her side, living with us was a significant adjustment for Jean. With four people in one house, her personal space was confined to a single bedroom and nearby bathroom. Even as our lifestyle and habitual patterns had to be realigned to fit her physical needs, her personal habits and activities had to be curtailed to fit our household patterns. Jean learned to let go of many freedoms she had while mistress in her own home. She could not have all her accustomed things around her in such limited space. She could no longer go where and when she wished. On the other hand, she was relieved of responsibilities she could no longer manage—marketing, food preparation, cleanup, laundry, scheduling appointments, and driving. Literally and metaphorically, this opened up more "breathing space" for her. There was a clear trade-off in freedoms as a result of being cared for in our home.

One of my greatest challenges was how to balance my own needs with my mother's, given our differing situations and personalities. Jean was a night owl and enjoyed staying up to read after supper. By the time I got home from a full workday, prepared dinner, helped with cleanup, returned a few phone calls, perhaps paid a bill, and got my mother ready for bed, it was always late by my internal clock. Adequate sleep was a casualty.

On weekends I had household chores and often preparation for event leadership. Even with John's help, I could only attend to my mother in a limited way. From my perspective, her *needs* were always met but her *desires* suffered—opening her boxes from storage in our attic, or organizing her massive stacks of health journals. Jean's way of distinguishing her needs from her wants didn't always match mine! At times, this created friction between us. I needed her to recognize that I was doing what I felt I could under the constraints of my own work, while she needed me to see how important some of these tasks were to her, given how short a time she had left to live. It often felt like an irreconcilable tension that left me frazzled and feeling guilty for not giving her more of what she wanted.

The most obvious challenge was physical stress, especially over the increasingly intense final eight months. As she got weaker, Jean needed help getting up to go to the bathroom at night and in the early morning. I learned to sleep lightly so as to hear the little bell she rang for help. John was a deep sleeper and found night awakenings more disruptive than I, so I usually handled these calls. Though Jean was small and not difficult to help, I struggled with exhaustion at every level. I have never been a high-energy person, so nightly interruptions of sleep brought me near to a breaking point physically. My challenges, of course, went well beyond the physical. Emotionally I grieved, preparing for her loss. Having lost my father to a train wreck when I was eight years old, my mother's role in my life was more central than any other with the exception of John's. It was an absolute *agony* to helplessly witness her body-wracking cough and struggle for breath—a struggle I felt empathically in my own body. With no time for my usual prayer practice, I felt spiritually depleted as well. I was hanging on by a thread, desperately trying to discern when Jean might be better served in a hospice residence. I yearned for freedom from the unyielding demands of her care, yet felt guilty for wanting a freedom that meant her death.

After one particularly frightening night of crisis, my mother and I agreed it was time for her to enter the hospice residence. This decision was an immense and immediate relief to me. Finally she would receive round-the-clock care from a medical team equipped to relieve her inflamed lungs and breathlessness. Yet even in those last three weeks of her life, I struggled with when and how long to visit as I tried to catch up with a vast backlog at work. Henri's words fit my experience:

> If the one we care for is a family member, we also may bear all the conflicting emotions of trying to support a loved one. On the one hand, there is the desire and willingness springing from our love for this person. On the other hand, our desire and willingness may be woven together with loneliness, resentment, guilt, and shame for unwanted thoughts and dreams of being free once more from the burden of care.[2]

One evening, a week after Jean entered the hospice residence, we received a call that she had taken a downward turn and might have only a few days to live. I called my brothers, who flew in the next day, and we took turns sleeping in her room overnight. Jean rallied with her three beloved children around her. She was excited and happy for four days. We prayed together and said all the things we wanted to say to each other. It was magical and profound. My brothers flew home and the vigil of death we had anticipated was postponed.

Professionals who work with the dying talk about what enables us to die well, including "relationship completion" and dealing with "unfinished business."[3] I experienced both in different ways with Jean. The days with my brothers at the hospice residence felt like a remarkable gift of relationship completion with our mother—remembering stories, expressing forgiveness, sharing deep gratitude and love, and saying our goodbyes. A week later, nurses again saw signs of the end. By now Jean's voice was so weak I could barely make out her words. She wanted to talk with John and me together about something. But while we were visiting her together, she was too groggy on morphine to talk, and that conversation never happened. She died early one morning before I could get to the residence. This left me not only with a sense of unfinished business, but guessing what that business might have been. For more than a year I felt guilty for not having made a more concerted effort to get John and me there at a time when she was alert. Her alertness could not be predicted, and my guilt was fairly irrational. Nonetheless it haunted me. Not only in the midst of caregiving, but after the death of our loved one, feelings of inadequacy and regret may linger. And this, after saying all we thought was needed a week earlier!

MY STORY WITH BAB

Little did I know that emotional conflicts would become even more acute in caring for my mother-in-law, whose story I turn to next. Bab cut a very different figure from Jean. My mother-in-law exuded a larger-than-life presence. Daunting in stature, vocal command, and emotional distance, she was once mistaken by our postman for English royalty! Her deafness reinforced a naturally loud voice with an adamant tone. Bab broke her hip just two months after Jean's death, so John and I had very little daylight between intense care situations. Although she made a remarkable recovery from hip surgery, Bab suffered poor balance, was prone to falls, and gradually went from cane to walker to wheelchair.

Mentally, Bab had long-standing if undiagnosed limitations. Like a child, she was a concrete thinker and counted even the simplest arithmetic on her fingers. She saw the world in black and white, judged by surface appearance, and suffered from attention deficit. Bab repeated family stories like a script—exactly the same words each time—and seemed oblivious to having told the same story the night before. This used to drive me utterly crazy, until I learned to tolerate the boredom and even ask questions about her family history. Emotionally Bab was distant, seeming unable to access her own feelings much less connect with ours.

Perhaps the greatest challenge was meeting Bab at her own level. For example, she was very anxious about dying. When I talked with her directly about death and drew out her own beliefs, she seemed able to express tentative trust. Yet if I offered her a very accessible book on facing death with hope, she invariably laid it aside for her preferred biographies and fiction. Bab was always reading, although it was never clear to us how much of it penetrated. In her final year of life she observed with ironic self-awareness, "I am not given to looking inward." John and I, accustomed to deep reflection on life's great questions, often struggled to find dinner topics she could share in. We found them in simple things: food, clothes, plants, cats, birds.

The physical demands with Bab were far greater than those with my mother. As she lost strength and mobility, it became increasingly difficult for me to manage, given her large bone structure and girth. Over the years, I contracted "frozen shoulder" three times from the strain of helping her stand and sit. In Bab's last few months of life, the intensity of my physical stress increased to the point that John and I seriously considered either investing in heavy lifting equipment for the home apartment or the nursing home option, which we considered a last resort. We were spared a final decision when Bab suffered a bad fall, was hospitalized, and died within a week from sepsis.

In her last few years, Bab's memory and ability to process information declined significantly. Clear communication became more challenging. Even with her hearing aid turned up, I had to speak very loudly to be heard. Being naturally soft-spoken, I found this hard to do without sounding angry—at least to myself. Even if I felt no frustration it seemed I was always shouting, which drained my energy! I learned to speak simply and slowly. While Bab often seemed like a child, she was not a child and readily detected condescension. Even when she expressed extreme anxiety and helplessness, John and I tried to find ways to calm her that kept her dignity intact. Threading our way between giving her emotional assurance, clear ground rules, and inviting her ownership in decisions she could still make was a real instruction in humility, patience, and discernment. As in the parenting of young children, complex interactions are often improvised on the fly without time to weigh options. We certainly didn't always get it right. In the final year we saw mild signs of paranoia; she was less trusting that we would make decisions in her best interest. It was painful to feel loss of trust from one we sincerely cared about.

OTHER STORIES

My personal experience is naturally limited, yet I learned from Henri that the most personal aspects of human life often evoke the most universal. We live by stories, each of which brings a unique element to the larger tapestry. Challenges in caregiving are immense and varied. Every story shines light on the big picture, adding color and shading that reveal deeper dimensions of the whole. It is time to widen the angle of our lens.

Stories make us more alive, more human,
more courageous, more loving.
—MADELEINE L'ENGLE

CHAPTER 2

Some of us manage care from a distance. My older brother and his wife have faithfully driven from Connecticut to Pennsylvania about one weekend a month for the past ten years as her parents needed increasing help in their declining years. Her mother died a few years ago, but her father—now 99 with fading memory—only recently stopped going to his law office every day. It was a tricky business to edge him, literally, out of the driver's seat!

When Sharon's father was mortally ill, she learned to release control and allow her mother to make decisions about her father's care that she herself would have made differently. Sharon's only sibling is a sister with moderate cognitive disabilities, whose care will come to her when her mother can no longer cope. Hers is a complicated, emotionally fatiguing family picture, involving a flight out of state every time she needs to offer support in person to her family members.

Some care stories are much more complex and intense. Emily was a typically developing child when at eight she began developing disturbing symptoms. At ten, she was diagnosed with a rare neurodegenerative disease. Within twelve months Emily could no longer walk, talk, or eat, although her mind was not damaged. She is now 24 years old. Her father, who holds a diplomatic post overseas and is gone for long stretches, has little involvement in Emily's care. Her mother, Lindsey, has taken almost exclusive responsibility for Emily's care these 14 years. For the last nine, Emily has been fed through a PICC line that delivers liquid nutrition straight to her heart. Lindsey must keep the feeding active for 19–20 hours a day. Her life is consumed with long stretches of intensive, medically complex nursing routines. Because Emily suffers terrible nerve pain, pain management is a constant feature of her care. At six feet in height, Emily is a great challenge for Lindsey to lift, but lift she must to get her daughter regularly repositioned in bed.

With her older son and youngest daughter gone from home, and her husband abroad, Lindsey is on her own with Emily's care. Recently the daytime hours of professional nurses helping in her home were expanded, just when Lindsey felt at the brink of complete exhaustion and despair. "I never fully realize how tired I am until something happens that brings relief to me, because my adrenaline just has to keep going and I have to keep rising to the occasion. When relief comes, I'm shocked at how overwhelmingly tired I am." Lindsey notes that friends and extended family members often don't fully understand what it's like to have your energies continuously available to one person in the inescapable confines of your own home. "I haven't had a bedroom for all these years," Lindsey muses. "My bed is right next to Emily's because she cannot be left for any period of time. She is monitored constantly, day and night, day and night. We've been on this treadmill for years now." Added to the direct demands of Emily's care is Lindsey's concern for her marriage. Her husband's current diplomatic post is in Africa. On long-distance calls, the contrast between the noise of embassy parties in the background and Emily's agony in the bedroom is stark. "I don't want to become bitter and resentful," Lindsey says quietly, "but it's hard. I need to be resurrected every day."

For those of us with less demanding situations, it is unimaginable how any one survives this level of intense, long-term caregiving. Yet Lindsey can say, "It is a raw, but rich life."

Lindsey's story offers a glimpse of how caregiving can stress a marriage. The challenges are sometimes more severe, as we see with Karen and her husband. The youngest of their four daughters, Hannah, was born with autism. Early in Hannah's life, there was a period of seven years when she didn't sleep for more than a few hours each night. While awake, she screamed non-stop. It was harrowing and exhausting for everyone. Karen's husband did not cope well with the stress and abandoned ship when Hannah was 11, leaving the entire family unsupported. "So there I was 24/7," Karen tells, "in the most real way responsible for everybody, and no one to help me." She somehow soldiered on as the lone parent for five years—forging ahead with very limited financial resources, growing more physically and emotionally exhausted by the day.

When Hannah was 16 and the older girls had left home, Karen finally succumbed to depression and anxiety: "I literally saw myself standing at the edge of a cliff, and fell over. I lost my mind for a time." For two-and-a-half years Karen spent most of her day in bed, unable to function beyond the effort of getting Hannah to school and picking her up. She shopped at a local drugstore for TV dinners because a market felt overwhelming. People were brought in to help with Hannah's needs and Karen was put on five different medications which, in her words, "kept me in a fog for two-and-a-half years." When at length she came off "the meds," she got in touch with her feelings: "I was so mad at my ex-husband," she exclaimed. "I was on my own for ten years, without support. I was soooooo mad at him!"

> *Resentment is a real option. Many choose it. When we are hit by one loss after another, it is very easy to become disillusioned, angry, bitter, and increasingly resentful. ... Resentment is one of the most destructive forces in our lives. It is cold anger that has settled into the center of our being and hardened our hearts.*
>
> —Henri Nouwen

The family repercussions of caring for a child with disabilities can be devastating. Thankfully, Karen recovered her bearings. Hannah is now in her mid-twenties and has come a long way with intensive one-on-one help. She is very bright—gifted in math, music, and language. It has been a long, hard road to gain understanding of Hannah's condition, support for her learning needs, and appropriate job options that fit Hannah's abilities and limitations as she moves through early adulthood. The challenges have been grueling.

NAMING HARD THINGS HONESTLY

It is important—emotionally and spiritually—to name the hardest feelings and experiences in our caregiving stories. Unless we can acknowledge and express these realities, we cannot allow them to be reframed and healed—one of the great works of the Spirit in us.

Here (italicized) are some hard feelings I can name. Over her last few years, I *yearned* for Bab to let go this earthly life—both for her sake and ours. I felt little guilt about this. The years of caregiving truly *felt interminable.* John and I joked privately that Bab was the "energizer bunny" who just kept going and going and going! My feelings were not merely self-centered: John and I had made many sacrifices—physical, financial, and emotional— over these years. We were deeply tired and had not had a week's vacation to ourselves in nine years. Hopes we had nurtured for a special anniversary trip to Europe had all gone by the wayside since Jean's heart attack in 2000. In many ways, I *felt deprived* of ordinary forms of relaxation that friends and family seemed regularly to enjoy: movie nights, dinners out, a weekend exploration of an interesting town—even just a few hours to curl up with a good book! I was *deeply envious* of friends whose Christmas letters described fabulous anniversary vacations in beautiful locales around the world. I felt John and I were missing out on some of the best gifts of life.

With far less reason than Karen, I could slip into *resentment* over what was lost in the years given over to caregiving. I was fortunate to have a very supportive husband, though his work consumed most of his week and he had less time than I to help directly with care. Still, John wanted to help as much as he could, evenings and weekends. And when my work took me out of town for days at a time, he faithfully picked up on home care for Bab beyond the hours of her daytime care aides. He was certainly supporting our family financially—especially in the last five years of his mother's life when I was only part-time self-employed.

Being more than ready for Bab to depart this life, *I felt relief* when she died. John, however, suffered *ample guilt* after his mother's death. I was away teaching and he felt responsible—it happened "on his watch." He felt that he should have seen Bab's true condition, even though trained medical professionals weren't seeing it. He *felt shame* that he, the only son, had let his mother down. I could not lift this burden from him, much as I tried. Guilt and shame are ruthless bedfellows!

Caring for others intensively or long-term evokes many hard feelings: fear for the safety and well-being of our loved one; anxiety over our adequacy to the task; fear of being judged; anger toward God, others, and ourselves; shame and guilt; physical and emotional exhaustion; isolation and loneliness; feeling unsupported or under-appreciated; grief at losing dreams of the life we had imagined; envy of those less burdened by care; frustration, even despair at limited time, energy, and financial resources; desperation at the relentlessness of care; relational stress with the loved one receiving care, or conflict with other family members involved.

The challenges are legion. If we understood fully from the outset the costs of our commitment to the role of caregiver, we might shrink back in fear and dismay. Perhaps it is a grace that when we find ourselves in situations we did not plan on, we take them on with a certain naïveté. As we grow into the full realities of care, we are given countless opportunities to let the challenges stretch and mature us.

Perhaps a year after Bab's death, I recognized her care as my "unchosen vocation." In a secular sense, vocation suggests the freedom to choose a path in life that fits our best gifts and heartfelt passion. This was not my experience in caring for my mother-in-law. Bab was not a person I would freely have chosen to develop an intimate relationship with. Yet in a spiritual sense, vocation is *God's call upon us*, and I was called to Bab's care by the circumstances of our lives. With time, patience, and growing awareness, I came to accept and even embrace that call. I could recognize some of its gifts with gratitude and marvel at an emerging sense of emotional connection, which I will describe in the next chapter.

> *Patience is a hard discipline. It is not just waiting until something happens over which we have no control ... Patience is not a waiting passivity until someone else does something. Patience asks us to live the moment to the fullest, to be completely present to the moment, to taste the here and now, to be where we are. When we are impatient we try to get away from where we are.*
> —HENRI NOUWEN

However—and this is important to hear—my struggle with the "unchosen-ness" of the call never entirely ceased. As the years of responsibility for Bab dragged on beyond any time frame we had imagined, I ever more desperately coveted freedom from the constraints of her care. More times than I care to recall, my patience wore thin, undermining my ability to be fully present. I yearned for an end to the stress. I craved time with John alone. The demands in those final years were increasing precisely as our energies were being depleted. Even adding more time for hired home aides, we could not afford enough hours to give us the respite we needed for replenishment. *The impact of caregiving is cumulative.* This is one of the most challenging aspects of caring long-term for those who are losing capacity.

Henri candidly acknowledges, "There is often a huge cost to the caregiver, and sometimes the care we give springs not from a well of love and altruism but from a bitter sea of resentful duty and obligation."[4] In my experience it is not an either-or situation. Conflicted feelings coexist! Within the space of ten minutes I could feel resentful duty when Bab's needs interrupted other important tasks or relationships, *and* authentic love while personally attending to her needs. Our human feelings and motives are a complex and shifting quicksilver.

About halfway through the eleven-year-long "interruption of my real ministry," it finally became clear to me that the manner in which I cared for Bab was in fact my primary spiritual practice for this season of life. If her care was at first a vocation by circumstance not choice, my task was to *make* it a free choice— to say Yes instead of resisting it. I am an ordained minister with a call to teach and write; I kept thinking I had more important contributions to make than giving Bab a shower, drying and dressing her, reconciling her checkbook, helping her remember buttons on the TV remote. But God was offering me an opportunity to use my time, energy, and relational gifts in ways that were more humbling and less exalted than I would have preferred. My obedience was to embrace this as a true vocation. Jesus' words to Peter at the end of John's Gospel capture something of how it felt to me: "I tell you most solemnly, when you were young you put on your own belt and walked where you liked; but when you grow old ... someone else will put a belt round you and take you where you would rather not go" (John 21:18, JB). Yet if I felt this way, imagine how Bab would have applied this passage to her life!

CHALLENGES FOR THE CARE RECEIVER

Being the person on the receiving end of care is full of hardship as well. As caregivers, how do we attend beyond the needs of physical or intellectual decline to the emotional and spiritual pain of those we care for? Henri speaks directly to some of these challenges:

> Important for us as caregivers to remember here is that it is embarrassing to be exposed in weakness and to need help. Having managed their own lives so easily for so long for both themselves and others, those who are ill or weak may find it humiliating to have to receive care and ask someone else to help them, especially if the one asked is already busy and occupied with important matters.
>
> Another very real sorrow for those receiving care is that it is not easy to wait—sometimes in pain—for someone to do for them what they can no longer do for themselves. It is bad enough for them to feel so fragile and so scared, but worse still to have to trust someone else—someone they may not know at all and who never knew them when they were strong. It can be humiliating to allow a stranger or even a family member to enter their intimate, physical, and private space. In other words, it is miserable for them to feel that they are the powerless one in the carer/cared-for relationship.[5]

Over the years I observed plentiful challenges for Bab. Some were external, like an uneven quality of care from home aides. Being stoical, Bab would often not tell us for weeks about an aide whose presence was less than helpful. On the other hand, she might lightheartedly complain that her caregivers were overeager to help her even with things she could still do for herself!

Largely, however, Bab's sufferings were matters of the heart. Like most who live to an advanced age, she had to let go much of the life she had known, including the independence she so cherished. Bab had lived abroad as a widow for 25 years, relishing her freedom. In coming to live with us she left behind a whole community of rich friendships, her beloved church, and the routines of life in a place she knew like the back of her hand. Transplanted to an unfamiliar setting, her world shrank dramatically. Although a few neighbors were gracious, including her in outings on special occasions, Bab felt they were more our friends than hers. Our small family and her daytime care aides became her primary social circle. She loved her little apartment in our home and claimed that she never felt lonely, but I could see the sadness in her eyes every time she received news of another friend's death—part of the increasing isolation that comes with a long life.

Slowly losing physical and mental capacities, Bab underwent the great stripping we call "the diminishments of age." Depending on others for even simple tasks took a toll on her sense of competency and self-worth. At times she was angry with herself for being "clumsy" or "stupid." At other times she seemed sadly bemused, surprised to have become someone she scarcely recognized. "How did I get to be like this?" she wondered aloud.

The younger we are the more people we need so that we may live; the older we become, the more people we again need to live. Life is lived from dependence to dependence.
—HENRI NOUWEN

The pain of feeling like a burden to John and me was expressed as "being useless." Bab loved to cook, and for many years it gave her great satisfaction to provide one or two meals a week for the three of us. When she could no longer cook, she felt she could make no further contribution to our life together. As a concrete thinker, Bab had trouble seeing any mutuality in our relationship after that. Her requests for help seemed mere imposition, unbalanced by any reciprocity from her side. I saw that, even in advanced age, having some recognizable contribution to make to the lives of others remains critical to our sense of self-worth and will to live.

With both of our mothers, I observed a frustration I call the "wait factor." Apart from central care routines or emergency needs, when Jean or Bab called on us for help we sometimes had to keep them waiting. The speed of our response depended on the importance of their requests in relation to competing responsibilities. The same situation faces those who wait on the response of nurses and aides in hospitals, nursing homes, or assisted care facilities. Being dependent as an adult is hard to accept, sometimes frightening, and often depressing.

The challenges of receiving care can be intense for people with severe disabilities or degenerative diseases. Judy was diagnosed with Parkinson's disease at age 20. A fetal tissue transplant has given her 20 years more of life. Yet without family to help, she is highly dependent on multiple home caregivers. One of her early challenges was simply accepting the fact that she needed help. "I'm not used to seeing myself as the incapacitated one," she admitted. Only as the disease progressed and her limitations became more apparent could she acknowledge that help was more than a luxury. Judy confides that her physical changes have been hard to accept: "You always want to appear at your best with others."

Needing substantial help from others involves losing a measure of control over your own life. Judy named some of the issues she has faced with caregivers over time. She needs two or three care aides a day and doesn't always know who will arrive at her door. While some are good, others are under-qualified with little altruistic motivation for the job. Judy has been taken advantage of: unauthorized use of her credit card by a caregiver purchasing personal groceries; items of clothing or jewelry stolen; even violations of Judy's physical safety, when she was struck. People requiring high levels of care are deeply vulnerable to physical and emotional abuse.

Often, however, the issues Judy struggles with involve exercising greater choice. Caregivers come with lists of things to accomplish, and may be more interested in checking off the list than in what Judy wants help with: "Sometimes they do not value what I ask them to do." Her caregivers are more concerned with her safety than she is. As a self-admitted risk-taker, Judy recognizes that she can be a handful for her caregivers to care for! Yet Judy desires to keep her mind and life as active as possible. She likes to get out when she can. She has hopes—in the time remaining to her—to support refugees with Parkinson's, or help children understand what it's like to function with disability. Judy wants to live her days as fully as possible, and not all care aides support that aspiration.

What does Judy value most in a caregiver? Willingness to relate to her as a full human being, not a list of care tasks; companions who respect her, feel some affinity for her, bring a sense of humor and a little fun into their daily life; aides who listen well and have a desire to understand her; who are willing to cook food she enjoys; who have the freedom to be flexible. In essence, Judy yearns for caregivers who value *being* as much as *doing*. "The key to meaning," she says with emotion in her voice, "is *bonding with others*." Judy's story reveals again that the core of caregiving is the quality and character of our relationships!

I trust that those of us engaged in care relationships do indeed take time to listen with an open heart to the needs and desires of those who receive our care. It can be useful to hear the voice of a strong-willed and vibrant person like Judy, whose experience helps us stay attuned to the challenges of care receivers.

In this chapter we have hinted at the other side of our caregiving paradox: that sorrows and joys are intertwined, that challenges and gifts can never be entirely separated from each other. It is to the gifts and joys we turn next.

The Gifts of Caregiving

SEEING AND CELEBRATING

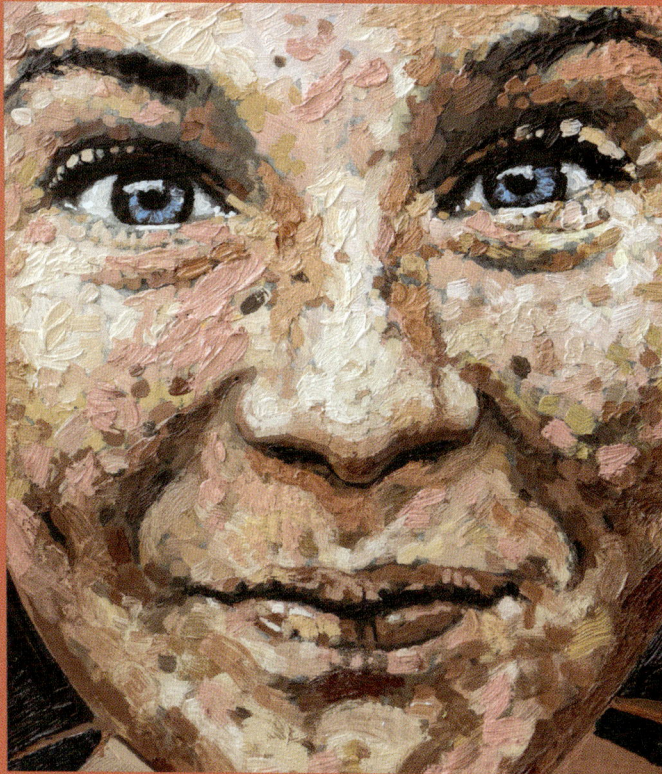

A ATTENDING TO STRESSES felt by those receiving our care reminds us of the central truth of *mutuality* in caregiving. We are vulnerable human beings on both sides of giving and receiving. No relationship is ever a one-way street, no matter how incapacitated the person receiving care may be, and reciprocity is real even if the relationship appears unevenly weighted. Mutuality becomes more meaningful as we recognize the *gifts* received while caring for others. Yes, care brings heartache and hardship, but it is also a sacred privilege. One of Henri's closest friends captures both aspects, describing these relationships as "tortuous and transforming"[1]—a remarkably apt phrase.

OUR BELOVEDNESS: THE GROUND OF GIFTS

As we open our hearts to the Spirit, we begin to see how much more we receive in giving than we may first recognize. The reason, spiritually speaking, is quite simple: Each of us is imprinted at our core with the divine image, however dim or distant it may seem. Deep in the heart of each person dwells an imperishable glory, freely given to us and cherished by our Creator beyond our wildest imagining! God loves us with an everlasting love not because we are "good" or even making progress toward goodness, but because we belong to a God who loves.

> *The most important thing you can say about God's love is that God loves us not because of anything we've done to earn that love, but because God, in total freedom, has decided to love us.*
> —HENRI NOUWEN

Henri never ceased to proclaim that we are all beloved children of God: "At the core of my faith belongs the conviction that we are the beloved sons and daughters of God. And one of the enormous spiritual tasks we have is to claim that and to live a life based on that knowledge."[2] Our belovedness does not depend on our status or accomplishments or wholeness. In the upside-down economy of Grace, the least among us—the sick and forgotten, the weak and vulnerable, the disabled and frail—are often precisely the ones God works through most powerfully. Here is how Henri framed it: "Every person is an unrepeatable expression of God's creative grace. God can minister through anyone, and often does so in and through the least, the little ones, the handicapped, the poor, the unimpressive."[3] Caregivers are called to recognize that the person receiving care is as dearly loved by God as we—even if that person is the crabbiest curmudgeon on the planet; even if that person lies on a bed in an unresponsive state day upon day; even if that person's behavior is difficult to understand or tolerate. These beloved ones of God are truly our teachers if we allow them to be—as many caregivers have discovered with time. Henri delighted to begin his talks with the theme of our belovedness. He would say, in essence, "Listen deeply to the voice of the great lover of souls. Hear that you are beloved. Then you can see that others are, too."

RECOGNIZING THE GIFTS OF CAREGIVING

It was easy to perceive the joys of caring for Jean. I was blessed beyond deserving to have a mother who in so many ways embodied unconditional love. Although strong-willed and never afraid to speak her mind, Jean was deeply wise, sensitive, and open. She listened well to others and to her own heart; I rarely hesitated to talk with her about anything. Her love for me drew out my responding love.

When my step-dad, who suffered from dementia, was placed in assisted care, my mother asked if she could live with us for what she surmised to be the last few months of her life. I had no reservations about taking her in, though it meant John and I would have both our mothers living with us for a time. I knew Jean's physical needs were acute, but my heart leapt at the opportunity to reciprocate in some small measure all the care she had given me over my lifetime.

Jean lived with us for 20 months, longer than expected. After a year, when she expressed sorrow to be a burden in our lives, I could candidly say: "Yes, there is a burden in your care, but even more it is a great joy to have you with us, and I wouldn't have it any other way! If I could go back and choose again, I would make the same choice." I did not deny that we felt a burden in caring for her. Jean could see my fatigue and was always an ace in detecting white lies! Yet my honesty about the hard side allowed her to hear equal truth in the happy side: my assurance that I *wanted* to be her primary caregiver at the end of her life, and found fulfillment in that choice because of who she was and what she meant to me.

I can identify several particular gifts we enjoyed in the mutuality that marks intimacy. Conversations of the heart arose amid daily activities that would not have occurred had I been visiting my mother in a care facility. Often they came in moments of intimate care: helping her get showered, dried, and dressed; sitting on her bedside before nestling her under the covers at night; massaging her legs and feet as she lay in bed. Communication emerged naturally in the course of caregiving itself, and feelings were shared as they surfaced. At night, when conversation subsided, she would remind me that it was late and I must be tired—that I had done enough.

We had leisure to deliberate about Jean's end-of-life decisions and desires in an unhurried way. Everything about her wishes was clear. She put her affairs in order, making sure I knew where her important papers were and what her financial position was.

We had many opportunities to say everything we wanted to each other. Each of us knew we were dearly loved by the other, and my mother understood how deeply I would miss her.

Jean had no fear of what lay on the other side of death. While she was not looking forward to the final act of dying, her faith was strong and her trust in the reality of the communion of saints was a blessing. I knew she suffered no needless anxiety, but rather carried a spirit of inner peace. Our shared faith was a great gift to me, especially when I felt anxious or grieved about her suffering. Henri wrote a book on "befriending" our death and making it our final gift to others. He raises some basic questions: "Is death such an absolute end of all our thoughts and actions that we simply cannot face it? Or is it possible to befriend our dying gradually and live open to it, trusting that we have nothing to fear?"[4] Without knowing Henri's language, Jean had deeply befriended her death. She would have answered No to the first and Yes to the second of these questions.

Above all we were appreciative of the precious gift of one another's presence. Jean had always been present to me, which made it natural for me to respond in kind. In our home, she was present for all our family celebrations—if only standing at the loft railing looking down, tethered to her oxygen tubes. With her presence came warmth, vitality, and her sardonic wit—bringing smiles and much-needed levity. I will never forget the last exchange between my mother and Bab, the day the ambulance came to take my mother to the hospice residence. Bab, never comfortable with finalities, put on an unconvincing smile and said, "Oh Jean, I hope we will see you back here again very soon!" Jean—who had to gasp for air every few words—retorted in her gravelly voice, "Well, don't hold your breath!" Bab caught neither the irony nor the gallows humor, while John and I barely contained outright laughter!

Since my relationship with Bab was complicated, it took time for me to recognize the gifts in her care. Her deafness—physical and emotional—alongside her cognitive limitations, made it hard to connect intellectually or spiritually. Like Henri's experience with Adam, our *understanding* of spiritual matters had little relevance for Bab. We had to *live* our spiritual life with her. Bab taught me to "walk the talk" since she couldn't "get" the talk.

For years, Bab literally stiffened if John or I embraced her. She seemed repelled by physical affection, blowing kisses from across the room—a perfect expression of emotional distance. But the more I learned about her stern upbringing and her father's harshness, the more I saw her inner wounds. She received little affirmation or warmth from her parents as a child and did not know her belovedness. Entering her room, I would sometimes hear her mutter to herself, "Winifred, you stupid girl." Harsh self-judgment rose up from the unhealed child in her heart.

Henri notes that it can be a "long and difficult passage into accepting to be beloved while in a weakened condition."[5] This is true, yet for people like Bab a weakened condition is not the source of uncertainty. She endured a lifetime of hidden vulnerability. Bab had taught Sunday school children about God's love but couldn't trust that love for herself. I began to recognize a tug in my heart to show her more tangible affection—to express that she was loved just for who she was. She needed concrete evidence, the very physical expressions of love she appeared determined to repel. I decided simply to plant a kiss on her cheek every time I said, "Good night." Before long, Bab showed clear signs of looking forward to that kiss. And if it appeared I might be about to forget, she would tap her cheek to remind me! This soon became an unalterable ritual—first just between the two of us, until gradually John was drawn in as well, much to my delight!

> *You were the beloved before you were born and you will be*
> *the beloved after you die. That's the truth of your identity ...*
> *You belong to God from eternity to eternity. Life is just an*
> *interruption of eternity, just a little opportunity for a few*
> *years to say, "I love you, too."*
> —HENRI NOUWEN

Over time, Bab began to believe me when I said—along with that kiss—"I love you, Bab." It was easier for me to show Bab tender gestures of love than it was for John, who grew up with the wounding effects of an emotionally distant mother. Freedom from the tangled web of family history was one of the great gifts in my role as daughter-in-law. It was an unexpected happiness that my freedom had positive ripple effects in John and Bab's relationship.

The trust that flowered between Bab and me paved the way for me to help her more as her physical needs grew. She entrusted me with her intimate care, and I recognized it as an opportunity to minister further to her through touch. Massaging Bab's arms, back, legs, and feet with a creamy, fragrant lotion after her shower was one of our sacred rituals. We engaged in face-to-face interaction—questions, responses, smiles, little jokes—just the simple pleasures of being together. The physical closeness brought us together emotionally, and quickened the growth of our love for each other. Henri addresses this mysterious dynamic with amazing spiritual depth in one of his journals:

> The bodily resurrection of Jesus is the most profound basis for the sacredness of all human flesh and the most compelling argument for reverencing all forms of life. ... Washing, dressing, feeding and supporting deeply handicapped people is a holy vocation when we know

that their bodies, like ours, are destined to share in the resurrection of Jesus.[6]

In her late years, Bab often thanked me for my care after I got her under the bed-covers. She was genuinely grateful, and I was glad for her willingness to express it. Her gratitude was a real gift to me—one that not every caregiver receives. I often responded by taking her hand and saying, "You are very welcome, Bab. I'm glad to help you in any way I can because I love you!" I meant it, and she knew it.

When Bab fretted about having no contribution to make to our family life, I reminded her how much she helped us in the past, and not just by cooking dinner. Part of our family story included her 14 years of effort to get compensation for her husband's property, lost after the Turkish invasion of Cyprus. That effort finally paid off and made it possible for us to build a home with a specially designed apartment for her final years. She had already made substantial contributions to our life! Remembering these truths helped assuage Bab's shame at feeling useless.

Like my mother, Bab expressed sorrow in being a burden to us. I would respond: "Yes, but a burden we have freely chosen because you are family and we love you. We each need to accept the circumstances we find ourselves in as our days unfold—and just live with all the love we have." I could help her accept that we were in this together by the grace of God—a perspective as helpful to me as to her.

Years ago Parker Palmer—a close friend of Henri's—observed, "Sometimes we don't think our way into a new way of living; we live our way into a new way of thinking." His words described precisely our path with Bab. Physical care was how she knew we loved her, and for me at least, the way I "lived into" loving her.

Accompanying our loved ones through caregiving will always entail struggle. Why imagine that we should achieve perfect harmony in these relationships? Life is messy, people are complex, feelings are confusing, truth is paradoxical—nothing comes in clean, straight lines. Yet this I can say truthfully: More than any other person, Bab taught me patience—along with a deep acceptance of human limitation and weakness, including my own. I slowly learned to accept her for who she was without feeling a need to change her. Bab had her own dignity and charmingly peculiar belovedness! She was wounded and anxious; yet, as Henri said, God can minister through anyone and often does so through those we least expect.

Bab was my unwitting teacher. She kept me humble by revealing me to myself—my reactions, unrealistic expectations, ego needs, fear and anger. In her maddening stubbornness, she showed up my inability to fix, change, or control others to my liking. Bab gave me plenty of grist for growth. She drove me daily to prayer and my need for the Spirit of grace.

In the last few years of her life, I prayed for eyes to see the face of Christ in Bab. It was a spiritual challenge to "see Christ in his distressing guise" (a favorite phrase of Mother Teresa of Calcutta). Yet Jesus teaches unequivocally: "I was sick and you took care of me;" and "just as you did it for one of the least of these … you did it for me" (Matthew 25:36, 40). It takes a faithful imagination to see the image of God in every person. There were times— unexpected moments breaking through the crust of ordinary perception—when God gave me eyes to see the hidden Christ in Bab's broken and beloved humanity. Those moments moved me to openhearted surprise and joy: I could glimpse Bab's inner beauty and courage, her gracious yielding to the changes of age, her remarkable perseverance, her acceptance of weakness and limitation. Then I could find light and laughter to share, and the two of us—giggling like young girls—would agree, "Better to laugh than cry!"

I ask you: What could be more precious than to see the face of our humble Lord shining in the flesh and bone of another human being, weak and imperfect as we all are? What better gift could there be in this world?

MORE STORIES OF GIFT

In the last chapter we met Emily and her mother, Lindsey. Emily is confined to bed and cannot talk, but her mind is alert. She understands perfectly what others say to her and responds through expressive eyes and facial demeanor. Her mother says Emily is tremendously insightful and has a good sense of humor. She loves music and knows Bible stories by heart. "They aren't just stories," explains her mother. "These were people who, in times past, had to live with very difficult circumstances, who often waited long years not knowing how things would turn out. Their lives reflect something of hers, and she needs to hear that she's not alone in this experience." Lindsey reads regularly to Emily. With favorite books like the Chronicles of Narnia, "the characters are family to her."

Lindsey names some of the gifts of caregiving she has known in a profoundly mutual relationship with her daughter.

Who nurtures who more? I don't know; it's very cyclical. We're always exploring new things together. The big question is what does it mean to live? I was always a sensitive, tender, compassionate person. Yet I would never have imagined being able to give to Emily the way I have been able to give to her, or her being able to give to me the way she gives to me. The big message is "There is always more, and always enough." We laugh together, we cry together. It's not like it's perfect all the time; when you're tired and when the pain goes on for days, we aren't at our best. However, I know that what we are living is extraordinary and is all a gift. She knows it too. If I can keep articulating to her in very specific ways the gift she is to me, those are the words of life that penetrate her and resuscitate her again and again. When it does that to her, it does that to me too.

Lindsey recounted a recent episode, after months of doctors failing to get Emily's pain under control. "In the middle of all her agony and anguish, when I was standing by her bed that night, the Spirit impressed on me to say: 'Your life doesn't just have purpose in *this* life. Your life will continue to have purpose and meaning when you have passed beyond this life.' That was all she needed to hear. Emily looked up at me and just *glowed*. That was her thank you. Her eyelids closed and she went to sleep, no medicine, and no pain anymore." This poignant moment speaks volumes about our souls and the meaning we seek at the deepest level of our being.

Karen, mother to Hannah, describes her growth in faith as one of the greatest gifts she has received through caregiving. Karen grew up believing she needed to be "productive for God." Hannah introduced her to God in a new way. As Karen tells it,

> I had this little person in my life who would never make a "meaningful contribution" to society. And yet I knew that she had incredible value to God. When I grasped this, I realized that God didn't require anything from me except to understand his tremendous love for me; love that would give me life in this situation if I would just depend on him for my next breath the same way Hannah did. I got a very different view of who God was, and stopped trying to perform. Best thing that ever happened to me!

If Hannah's gift to Karen was a new way of relating to God, God also gave Karen a new way of seeing Hannah. When Hannah was young, Karen confessed, "I looked at my autistic child as a mistake, like somehow God missed something. I felt hopeless, thinking, 'This child is broken and there is no fix.'" In the midst of agonizing difficulties with a child unable to communicate, Karen heard God speak in her heart: "You see your daughter as flawed. But she is made in my image, and is perfect in my eyes. You need to learn to see her as I do." This message changed everything, giving Karen hope and a sense of purpose. Hannah was *supposed* to be here just as she was. She was not a shameful thing to be hidden away, but a person to be understood and brought as fully as possible into the human community. Like all parents, Karen could proclaim, "I want her to achieve everything she's capable of achieving!" With her mother's persevering support, Hannah has indeed achieved beyond all expectation.

Just as Henri experienced a role reversal with Adam, Karen experiences Hannah as her teacher: "I'm challenged every day with patience, kindness, tolerance. When she asks me the same thing the eighth or eighteenth time, I'm reminded that I can answer with gentleness and compassion, I don't need to lose my temper. I am not 100 percent successful in that, for sure, but I get to practice every single day! It's not so much doing the best I can as *being* the best that I *am*—which is a person having the nature of Christ in me. I remind myself who I really am. Everything that Hannah needs from me comes from Christ within me."

Remember, this is the mother who suffered from depression for years, and who—after coming off medications—came face-to-face with her fury at the husband who abandoned her. After struggling for some period of time with rage, Karen experienced an interior conversation with the Spirit in which it became clear to her that the Lord had been "father" to Hannah and "husband" to her. She acknowledged that God had sent just the right people into her life and opened doors for Hannah when Karen couldn't lift her head from a pillow. God had provided for all their needs.

"Why, then," the Spirit asked, "do you want to exact a pound of flesh from your mortal husband?" After this, Karen was able to call and forgive her ex-husband, releasing him from shame. "I continue to heal to this day," she affirmed.

There is so much in life that we don't sign on for. Yet the most stringent struggles may bring the most light. Two professors have coined the phrase "post-traumatic growth" to describe *positive psychological change* experienced as a result of coping with highly challenging circumstances.[7] Karen and Lindsey know by experience that as we allow ourselves to grow through the immense challenges put before us, they bring with them a much richer life experience. They would understand Henri perfectly when he writes, "People who have come to know the joy of God do not deny the darkness, but they choose not to live in it. They claim that the light that shines in the darkness can be trusted more than the darkness itself and that a little bit of light can dispel a lot of darkness."[8]

A few final perspectives on the gifts of caregiving come from Vanessa, whose 14-year-old son Charlie has physical and intellectual disabilities. We have looked at the negative family impacts of coping with a special needs child, stresses that can tear a marriage apart and strain the whole family. Yet there is another side to the story: Vanessa and her husband, Trey, work hard to make joint decisions about Charlie's care and education, even if they start off on different pages. "For very different reasons we both had a sense that *our* relationship needed to be at the core of the family," Vanessa explains. "As long as Trey and I are together, we can do anything." Vanessa's confidence in the strength of their relationship has born fruit in "a deeper and more trusting marriage—a different level of intimacy with another person than I would ever have imagined possible." The challenges of life can strengthen as well as weaken our closest relationships.

Much depends on our choices and in a marriage, those choices must be held by both partners.

As an academic, a second gift Vanessa identifies in her caregiving is a clear understanding that the brain is not equivalent to the soul. Charlie's intellectual disabilities have opened her eyes to this insight: "Your brain is not the source of human identity or humanity itself. I could have lived my whole life thinking: 'This is where Vanessa lives.' It is part of where I live. It is not what makes you a person or where your soul is. It is not why God loves you."

Those last words lead to the third gift Vanessa names. "I have always struggled with perfectionism," she confesses. "But I love Charlie and do not care whether he is perfect or not. That helps me think about how much God loves me, and therefore how I might imagine loving and caring for myself. I am still working on this. It is really about getting what grace is—that it is not earned. That is a huge, huge gift!" Perhaps Vanessa's honest struggle with perfectionism reminds us that we never achieve perfection in our life or our caregiving; we are *wounded* healers.

GIFTS FROM THE PERSPECTIVE OF CARE RECEIVERS

Receiving care, especially from those who love us dearly, comes with many gifts. My mother was certainly aware that her remaining life was extended perhaps ten-fold when we took her into our home. Instead of expending what little energy she had caring for a husband with dementia, she was freed to receive our care for her. She had the joy of being with one of her children on a daily basis, which meant the world to her. Jean felt deep appreciation for the time she was in our care, and reciprocated with loving generosity in every way she could.

Bab learned to *allow* us to love her, not merely to give dutiful care. She let her emotions be touched, and found small ways to respond in kind. Eventually she came to accept that our love for her did not depend on her "useful contributions," which in turn brought her the gift of greater self-acceptance. At the same time, our care for her became more emotionally satisfying to us as she received our love.

Care receivers give us *the gift of their vulnerability.* Each of our mothers embodied this beautiful insight, which Henri articulated this way:

> Our weakness and old age call people to surround us and support us. By not resisting weakness and by gratefully receiving another's care we call forth community and provide our caregivers an opportunity to give their own gifts of compassion, care, love and service. As we are given into their hands, others are blessed and enriched by caring for us. Our weakness bear fruits in their lives.[9]

Donna, the mother of a high-needs child named Nicholas, expressed vividly the delight of loving care that can be evoked by another's vulnerability and need:

> We *want* to give care. Not only is the right thing to do, but it gives us great pleasure and fulfillment to be able to look after the people we love. Just to bathe them and see them all clean and shiny, and to wrap up somebody you love. I always put the towels in the dryer to make sure they are nice and warm! You just love being able to give that comfort; it is so deeply satisfying.

Judy could acknowledge that she had likely given gifts to her caregivers: "I think I have given them courage," she mused, "maybe the will to put extra effort into something and not just do it carelessly. I've probably created patience in them because I have been such a pain in the neck sometimes!" And what were the gifts she had known in being a recipient of care? "Definitely more tolerance of myself; more acceptance of my limitations;

and willingness to ask for help. I've learned patience, and how to be gracious in receiving help."

A CLOSING STORY: FROM DARKNESS TO LIGHT

I conclude this chapter with a story from an extraordinary young man—a care receiver for nearly two decades—who died just recently. His words knit together the most profound challenges of human life with the greatest gem of God's gift to us, and reveal in short compass the journey of a soul from darkness to light. The young man's name was Reid, a deep and gifted soul, who fell from a roof at age 18 and lived as a paraplegic the rest of his days. Here is how he tells the story:

> I was watching a preview for the movie that chronicles the story of 33 Chilean miners trapped underground for 69 days. I began hearing the song, "Say Something." Part of me cringed as Nate Ruess began singing, "Say something, I'm giving up on you," because I'd heard the song played over and over again on the radio, and what I wanted to tell Mr. Ruess was, "Here's something, I've had enough of you." But another part of me heard something different. This part of me began listening to the song as if for the first time, and suddenly it was no longer a plaintive ballad about a man and a woman breaking apart, but the solitary voice of a lost soul giving up on God.
>
> I watched the 33 men trying to make sense of their captivity under a mountain in darkness, and when I heard Mr. Ruess's voice wail, "Say something, I'm giving up on you" what I heard was the voice of my own soul. I listened to the singer's voice wail … and I wailed right along with it, using that voice that is exhausted with trying to make things work, trying to keep hope alive, begging for nothing more than a response to its striving through a life that can seem one long, drawn out dark

night of the soul. Before I knew it I was weeping, weeping so hard that my body started shaking ... In my 36 years on this planet I have endured so much suffering.

I'm much like those coal miners trapped in the dark under a mountain of unknowing. I wonder if my prayers are being heard, and if the words I pray are right. What I've come to decide is that it's not the quality of one's prayer that makes the difference. What it all comes down to is having the courage to stand alone in the dark ... under one's own private mountain of suffering, and to realize that one cannot stay there long, if at all, without love. Go, stand under your mountain, feel yourself disappear against the burden that you carry, and know that you are a part of a greater good ..."[10]

The friend to whom Reid sent these words preached at his memorial service, saying, "Reid didn't 'believe' in Jesus ... he *knew* Jesus, the Jesus *'nailed to his predicament,'* as the songwriter Leonard Cohen put it. And, as best he could, Reid *followed* Jesus, the Compassionate One ... the Wounded One ... the Risen One."[11] A month before his death, Reid posted these words on Facebook:

I used to be so angry all the time—angry about being in a wheelchair, being in pain, being misunderstood. Now ... I feel nothing but subsumed in a constant state of being blessed, despite the chair, the pain, and the anger ... that has, for the most part, dissolved. It has taken me 37 years to reach this attitude of genuine blessedness. ... I am so very blessed. You are so very blessed. Realize this ... and carry it with you into the unflinching father of the Prodigal Son.

Henri's voice resonates right alongside Reid's—knowing Jesus as the wounded, compassionate One, knowing anguish and anger, knowing how these can be transfigured by grace to genuine blessedness. The father of the Prodigal Son was Henri's central image of the tender, persevering love of God—for himself and for us all. Moreover, Henri saw that once this love is deeply received, it is what we are called to embody: "What I do know with unwavering certainty is the heart of the father. It is a heart of limitless mercy ... I now see that the hands that forgive, console, heal, and offer a festive meal must become my own."[12]

Perhaps our hearts, too, are singing with Reid's and Henri's. Then again, we may be so tired or discouraged that the blessings of our situation largely escape us. It is difficult to absorb gifts when we are exhausted and drained. So we turn in the final chapter to our need for realistic self-care and spiritual practice.

The Sustenance of Caregiving
SELF-CARE AND SPIRITUAL PRACTICE

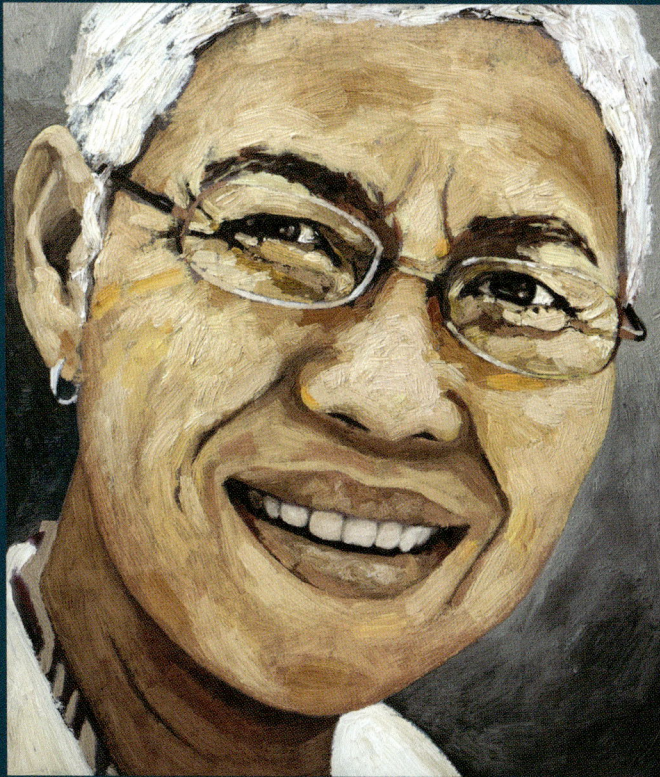

C AREGIVING IS A COMPLEX MIX of challenge and gift, exhaustion and fulfillment, grief and joy. We enter the fray with a range of motives—necessity, love, duty, service—that mix and shift over time. It is precisely over time that one question surfaces with growing insistence: How will our caregiving be sustained? "Sustainability" is now a central concept in relation to our planet. How do we live on this earth, with its finite and vulnerable resources, in a way that can be sustained for generations to come? The same question applies to each of us personally: With our finite time and energies, our vulnerable minds and bodies, how do we live out our care responsibilities in a sustainable way over the time that may be required of us?

This question lies behind every form of self-care. We are inevitably pulled in what feel like opposite directions between giving our energies to the care of others and taking time for adequate self-care. How, we wonder, can a realistic balance be achieved between two necessities in constant creative tension?

THE TENSIONS OF SUSTAINABLE CARE

For centuries, Western culture has burdened us with the notion that caring for ourselves is somehow selfish. Perhaps you are familiar with this formula—"Love God first, then others, and last of all yourself"—interpreted as humility. But if we think of self-love as last and least in importance, in practice it is easily lost. Henri's friend, Parker Palmer, offers a healthier and more realistic perspective: "Self-care is never a selfish act—it is simply good stewardship of the only gift I have, the gift I was put forth on earth to offer others. Anytime we can listen to true self and give the care it requires, we do it not only for ourselves, but for the many others whose lives we touch.[1]

When we are exhausted, the care we offer others suffers as well. And God does not require us to ruin our health to prove our love! Jesus models balance when he withdraws from the crowds to take time apart for prayer and inner renewal.

Self-care is a tender topic for caregivers. Lindsey acknowledges, "It's so hard to hear, 'Take care of yourself.' It's like someone telling a person who is already completely overwhelmed that there's one more thing they need to do!" Donna is in total agreement: "How many times are we told to take a bubble bath! The advice is in lieu of real support for caregivers. It just feels like an exercise in shaming. If we don't keep ourselves fit, it's *our* fault if we fall apart. This is not an invitation to extended families or community to befriend those of us giving care in our homes. The expectations just further isolate us." Lindsey observes that urgings to "care for yourself" often come from those close to her—husband, parents, or siblings who are not in a position to help with actual daily care—expressing their anxiety for her well-being. Without intending to, they project their fears onto Lindsey, one more weight for her to carry!

Yet despite their sensitivity to others' unrealistic expectations and fears, Lindsey and Donna well understand how crucial self-care is—simply to *survive* years of intensive home care for children with serious disabilities. The same can be said for those of us who care for spouses with Alzheimer's, or aged parents with deteriorating physical abilities. When we are in the trenches of long-term or sustained intensive care of others, self-care of some kind is not simply optional.

BROAD SELF-CARE PRACTICES

Michelle O'Rourke, a palliative care nurse with expertise on end-of-life matters, brings a helpful frame to this issue: "Self-care is an intentional way of living where our values, attitudes and actions are *integrated into our day-to-day routines*. It is not one more thing to add to our overflowing to-do lists, and is as much about letting go as it is about taking action."[2] Her realism is a breath of fresh air to overburdened caregivers!

Both Donna and Lindsey have discovered this truth for themselves. Donna has been experimentally re-thinking self-care: "What if every caring action we perform for somebody else could be an opportunity to do something for ourselves too?" She offers examples: "When I get someone a cup of tea, make myself a cup as well. If I feel cold, I put a sweater on my son—why not on me too? It means being mindful about how to care for yourself even as you care for another." Donna takes her thoughts a step further: "Can these simple shifts in awareness and behavior become an opportunity for deepening companionship? Doing *with*, rather than just doing *for*?" Donna is reframing simple acts of serving in a way that moves us toward a more conscious sense of mutuality, along with greater ease and enjoyment in the care relationship.

Lindsey would agree: "I try to include Emily in as many things as I can. Music works well for both of us." Lindsey plays songs from YouTube or brings an instrument to play by Emily's bedside; together they are nurtured by the soothing and refreshing power of music. Scripture and prayer are also central to Lindsey's spiritual self-care. Sometimes she attends to them in precious stretches of solitude, but she also reads the Bible and shares prayer with Emily. Notice that this gives Emily a way to participate in *her own self-care* at an emotional and spiritual level.

Donna integrated self-care into her family life in other natural ways. It was important for everyone in her family to know that she had expectations for civility and loving behavior, including their nurture of her. "Even Nicholas," she laughed. "I would say to him, 'I need a hug' or 'I know you have a lot to give the world, and the world includes me.' I refused to be invisible to those I was looking after." Donna's attitude is not only a healthy expression of self-respect, but also affirms the capacity of everyone in the family to be thoughtful, which helps generate their own self-respect.

When thinking through self-care, take into account who you are and what feeds you. Lindsey has engaged in many forms of self-care that fit her personality and needs: "I am a monk in disguise, so I retreat to my inner monk." For years she has been telling Emily's story on a CaringBridge website, often writing on a daily basis. "It gives me a place to process some aspect of the day," she says, "and that helps to keep me going." Because family and friends can respond to her journal entries on the website, this practice also helps her feel supported and connected to a wider community. Lindsey decided this year "that I needed to have a look at who I really am, and the things that make me who I am: letter writing and calligraphy—doing things by hand as opposed to the computer. I'm trying to branch out into artwork and photography, even poetry."

Interior reflection and creativity are nourishing to Lindsey's spirit. For you, it might be something quite different. In the years of my caregiving, getting out into the freshness and beauty of Creation was essential to my wellbeing. I could literally feel my depleted energy being replenished as I walked and breathed, absorbing the peaceful vitality of the natural world.

Michelle O'Rourke suggests that two of the most helpful questions you can ask yourself are: "Who holds you?" and "What refreshes you?" She has much to offer in the area of practical self-care for caregivers stretched to their limits. Here are some of her suggestions:[3]

- Take stock of what's on your plate. Prioritize; delegate; be selective.
- Find time for yourself every day—quiet, unplugged time.
- Identify what refreshes you and build it into your schedule
- Enjoy nature and the arts.

- Enjoy family and friends.
- Keep a sense of humor.
- Remember to play!
- Reflect on what you have given and received.
- Tend to your spiritual needs—cultivate an inner life.

You cannot do all these things every day, but together they offer a range of self-care practices that bring balance and renewal to your life. The first point is critical; setting even a few boundaries can open up much-needed space for self-care. Start with these questions: What care tasks do you *not* want to give away? What support tasks could others do? There are likely people in your life—neighbors, friends, extended family—who wish to offer help but don't know how. Donna suggests you choose three things you typically do in a week that you would love to give to someone else: yard work? grocery shopping? light housekeeping? Ponder: Who is in your literal or metaphorical "neighborhood?" What are others interested and gifted in? How might you give them a chance to support you?

> *No, we shouldn't try to care by ourselves. Care is not an endurance test. We should, whenever possible, care together with others.*
> —HENRI NOUWEN

The danger of neglecting sufficient self-care is *burnout*. Henri describes burnout as "giving without receiving." He makes several points on avoiding burnout as a caregiver:

- Look for the blessing of God in the poverty and dependence of those for whom you care, and recognize the gifts you receive in offering care.
- It is important not to be alone in caregiving, and to be aware of your limits.

- Realize when you need "time out" and don't feel guilty about it.
- It is important to be cared for yourself—who holds you?
- Trust that when you leave, your presence will continue.
- To be a good caregiver is to be really present.[4]

Regarding the final point, Henri notes that the most difficult thing is to be present but only half there—to be present without wanting to be, which leads to resentment. In my experience, being physically present without wanting to be resulted in care that was unsatisfying on both sides of the partnership. Inhabiting neither "here" nor "now," I was impatient, busily efficient with tasks, closed to deeper interaction, and frustrated by not being where I wanted to be. I've no doubt that Jean and Bab were fully cognizant of my mood and that it colored their own frustration at being dependent on my care! The point is that to resist being fully present in our care relationships adds a level of needless fatigue. As we allow ourselves to dwell in the "here and now" of care, stress is actually reduced.

When burnout is unrelieved we end up with "compassion fatigue," which Michelle describes as "profound emotional and physical erosion that takes place when helpers are unable to refuel and regenerate." Signs include:

- Becoming cynical or defensive; not enjoying work.
- Physical aches, pains, dizziness, difficulty sleeping, immunity impairment.
- Anxiety, depression, numbness, withdrawal; difficulty concentrating; feeling detached, apathetic, overly sensitive.[5]

These danger signs should prompt us to seek help. We are interdependent beings, not built to get through life on our own. Our individualistic culture promotes the myth of solitary heroes or heroines, triumphing alone against all odds. This is not, however, the message of our faith. We are created for community, to "bear one another's burdens, and in this way fulfill the law of Christ" (Galatians 6:2). When family and friends cannot offer adequate help, pastors, therapists, spiritual directors, and faith communities are available for support. It is crucial to learn when to ask for help, and to let ourselves receive help when needed. Here is the voice of writer and researcher Brené Brown urging us to let go "the myth of self-sufficiency":

> One of the greatest barriers to connection is the cultural importance we place on "going it alone." Somehow we've come to equate success with not needing anyone. Many of us are very reluctant to reach out for help when we need it ourselves. It's as if we've divided the world into "those who offer help" and "those who need help." The truth is that we are both.[6]

What does it mean to live in the world with a truly compassionate heart, a heart that remains open to all people, at all times? … When we are asked to listen to the pains of people and empathize with their suffering, we soon reach our emotional limits … But God's compassionate heart does not have limits. God's heart is infinitely greater than the human heart. It is that divine heart God wants to give to us so we can love all people without burning out or becoming numb.
—HENRI NOUWEN

REALISTIC SPIRITUAL PRACTICES

Given our limited time and energy, what spiritual practices are realistic for us as caregivers? Many classic practices require time set apart from ordinary activity. Centering Prayer asks for 20 minutes in silence twice daily; Spiritual Reading (*lectio divina*) takes at least 10–15 minutes, more if we add journaling; Intercessory Prayer lists can get so long they invite immediate procrastination!

The practices suggested here are selected to fit the realities of caregiving. They can help lighten our load by releasing heavy emotions, opening up limited perspectives, attuning our listening skills, and simplifying our prayer life. As with self-care, choose the spiritual practices that suit your circumstances and nourish your heart.

1. HONEST LAMENT

Before we can fully embrace the most difficult circumstances in our lives, we need to lament them. Scripture gives us permission to express the full range of human emotions. We see this in the book of Job and perhaps most fully in the Psalms, where praise and grief, joy and sorrow, contentment and fury contend with each other on every page—sometimes in the same psalm.

When we suffer, crying out in pain and anguish is natural. We clench our fist and utter our unanswerable "Why?" questions. Like Jacob at the Jabbok, we strive mightily with God through the night of our incomprehension, and perhaps come away with a permanent limp! (see Genesis 32:23–32). The struggle is necessary in coming to terms with suffering. As we wrestle with fear, anguish, fury, and desire for control, we are engaged in the grieving process—grieving a way of life we no longer have, or hopes and expectations that cannot be, or a terminal diagnosis for one who is dear to us. When we are brutally honest about the feelings we actually have, we can we offer them up—a living sacrifice—for the transformation only God can bring.

We could see this in a three-step process: First we let ourselves *feel our feelings*, taste them fully. This happens at a gut level— nonrational and preverbal. Feelings are raw, manifesting in our bodies as tension, tears, groans, or rising blood pressure. Second, we *recognize and name our feelings* for what they are—fear, anger, sorrow—and give them voice. Here the mind comes into play—seeing, understanding, and expressing. Finally, we *release our feelings* to the One who transcends them. It is a motion of surrender that spares us from getting stuck in our feelings and helps us look to the spiritual dimension of our lives.

Each part of this process is crucial to integration and healing. There are no shortcuts.

1. When we refuse to allow our feelings because they are painful or scary, what we repress moves deep into the shadows of our consciousness where it grows scarier and leaks out in unpredictable ways over time.

2. When we don't clearly see, name, and express our feelings, they remain a muddled mass just below the surface of our lives, generating confusion and blocking our energies. To "express" feelings literally means to "get them out." A healthy expression of feelings will be honest without harming others.

3. When we do not move to the stage of surrender—releasing our anguished or angry feelings to God—these emotions cannot be cleansed, healed, and reintegrated into our mature humanity. Jesus embodied our mature humanity. It is good news that as beings made in the divine image, we are destined by grace, ultimately, to grow into that maturity (2 Corinthians 3:17–18).

One of the most helpful practices we can turn to is "Praying the Psalms"—in this case psalms of lament. Select a psalm that expresses strong emotions of sorrow, anguish, incomprehension, or rage against "enemies" (enemies can be understood as what we are at war with in our own divided hearts). Among many psalms to select from, here are a few to consider: Psalm 13 ("How long, O Lord?"); Psalm 22 ("My God, why have you forsaken me?); Psalm 42 ("My tears have been my food day and night"); Psalm 69 ("Save me, O God, for the waters have come up to my neck.");

Psalm 77 ("Has God forgotten to be gracious?"); Psalm 88 ("O Lord, why do you hide your face from me?"). Perhaps only a few phrases or stanzas will speak to your life. Let the psalmist's cry resonate in your own weary, wounded soul. Personalize the ancient words, bringing your experience and feelings to it. You may paraphrase an existing psalm, or simply write your own from scratch. Here is a sample paraphrase of Psalm 13:

> How long, O Lord, must we keep this up? Forever?
> How much longer can I take the stress, the unknowing, the endless care?
> How much longer must I endure watching her suffer and shrivel by inches?
> My soul cries out within me for help and comfort!
> Look and answer me, O Lord my God!
> Give me some hope, or I will sleep the sleep of death soon myself.
> I put my trust in your saving help and love, O Lord.
> Do not abandon me!

2. REFRAMING

Many practices can sustain our caregiving that do not require stretches of time apart. One of the most helpful is to reframe our experience. As we go through life we turn it into a story, creating an internal narrative based on our perceptions and assumptions. We are largely unaware of these deeply held assumptions and the interpretations that follow them. Gaining new perspective can give us a different frame of reference, and thus a new story line.

I put a different frame around Bab's emotional distance when I began to see it as an expression of her fear and awkwardness, instead of seeing her as incapable of affection. We so easily misinterpret another person's thoughts and feelings. When I reinterpreted Bab's lack of warmth as a wound of deprivation, I could change my behavior toward her, which in turn drew out her affection and changed the dynamic between us. When I prayed to see Christ in Bab, I was asking God to put a new frame around my perception, to shift the lens through which I saw "reality."

Henri used to get frustrated by what he felt were constant interruptions of his work from phone calls or students knocking on his door. One day, he realized that "the interruptions" were *his* work! This reframing of his experience significantly reduced his frustration levels. The parallel for me was the moment I realized that the character of my care for Bab *was* my spiritual practice in that season of life. The reframing lifted my anguish over being unable to spend time in extended prayer and journaling. When Karen heard God say, "Hannah is perfect in my eyes and you need to see Hannah as I do," it allowed Karen to see her daughter's full humanity and rightful place in the world. This new lens not only re-energized Karen's hope, but redirected the ways she could advocate for Hannah's inclusion in public life.

In what ways might we change the frame on our caregiving? Perhaps just seeing this responsibility as a mission—a true calling of God—would make all the difference. Even if it feels like an "unchosen vocation," would freely embracing it change the frame? How might it change our view if we thought of our care receivers as souls who are offering themselves to us, in great vulnerability, for the sake of our own spiritual growth? Henri asked many reframing questions. Here is one: "Can you choose to live your losses, not as ways to resentment, but as ways to freedom?"[7] Judy, facing further decline with Parkinson's, speaks beautifully to the centrality of our choices: "Remember, you are the source of your own experience. Life isn't what it hands you, it's how you handle it. You will get much more from life by being positive than negative." Does Judy's hard-won wisdom resonate with you?

Jesus was always changing our frame on life—urging, inviting, exhorting us to see from the perspective of God's kingdom. The whole Sermon on the Mount is a reframing of reality, and the Beatitudes flip our ordinary assumptions on their head!

Here is a frame-changing meditation on the story of Simon of Cyrene, conscripted into carrying Jesus' cross when Jesus had no strength to carry it further:

> The cross of Jesus appears in many forms: Whenever you are the one who has to care for an aging parent because of circumstance; whenever you are the parent of a handicapped child, asked to do things ordinary parents aren't; whenever you're the one whose life is disrupted by unwanted circumstance, you are Simon of Cyrene helping Jesus carry the cross. The drama enfolded Simon and forced him to play an unglamorous, self-effacing, but needed role. His own agenda and plans had to be sacrificed and no doubt his response was less than fully enthusiastic. Yet this unplanned, humble service became the most important thing he ever did. Pure earthly accidents often make us responsible for what is divine and they conscript us to our real work.[8]

3. HOLY LISTENING

Listening becomes a spiritual practice when we discover it as sacred ground. Caregiving is a tremendous opportunity to learn how to listen more deeply to ourselves, to others, and to God. Natural ways of listening to ourselves are also important expressions of self-care: paying attention to what our bodies cry out for, like water or rest; listening to our feelings; noticing what we need to process mentally each day; tuning into our desire for support from family, friends, or faith communities.

Listening well to others involves a learning curve for most of us. An ancient philosopher once said, "We have two ears and one mouth so that we can listen twice as much as we speak."[9] But we tend to listen with one ear while the other is busy hearing the response we are formulating in our head! Real listening asks us to relinquish our agenda and simply open to what the other wants to communicate. Human communication is scarcely a matter of mere words. Caregiving with an intellectually disabled child, or an elder whose dementia is erasing neural pathways to words, gives us practice in learning a larger language. Donna speaks directly to this by-product of looking after Nicholas:

> Having a child who is non-speaking, I became a very good listener on many different levels—a full body, full mind, full spirit listener. You have to watch his body language very carefully as you listen to his verbal cues. You have to watch where his eyes are going, and put it all together to figure out what he's saying. That kind of listening has made me more deeply aware of how to be in this world with other people generally.

The most basic and powerful way to connect with another person is to listen. Just listen. Perhaps the most important thing we ever give each other is our attention .... A loving silence often has far more power to heal and to connect than the most well-intentioned words.
—RACHEL NAOMI REMEN

Listening fully to others is a sacred art, one of the deepest expressions of human care we have at our disposal. Sometimes it is the gift we most need, for to be truly heard is not only comfort but affirmation of our dignity and value. In caregiving we often don't know how to be of greatest help, especially when we can do little to alleviate another person's suffering. It is freeing to

discover that simply being a listening presence to our care
receiver may be the best gift we can offer.[10]

4. SIMPLE PRAYERS

What makes listening a holy act is recognizing divine presence
at the heart of everything—whether in hearing our inner world
more clearly, or in listening openly to another, or in turning our
attention directly to the Holy One. Listening to God in the midst
of daily challenge and gift is the crux of prayer. Some ways of
prayer are easy to integrate into ordinary life.

Breath Prayer. Sometimes we need to stop what we're doing
long enough to breathe deeply and center attention at the core
of our being. The Holy Spirit resides at the center of who we
are—an image of our inmost heart. We know intuitively how
to still our busyness and "center down." Paying attention to our
breath puts us in touch with what gives life. God is Spirit. The
Hebrew word for *spirit* and *breath* is the same. God sustains us
with holy breath in each moment. We can simply absorb this
gift, feeling the presence and energy of divine life in our own
breath. The life force revealed in breath can also bring us a sense
of sustaining love. Imagine filling your heart and lungs with
God's love! This practice takes very little time, yet can bring deep
refreshment, calm, and joy.

Another way to practice "Breath Prayer" is to form a very short
prayer phrase in two parts that moves rhythmically with in-
breath and out-breath: "Holy Spirit, fill me." "Gracious God, heal
my heart." "Lord Jesus, have mercy." "Oh Lord, give me patience."
Take a little time to find a phrase that fits your life. Then spend
a few minutes breathing this prayer before you rise from bed,
breathe it as you shower or gaze out a window, call it to mind in
times of stress, offer it up before drifting off to sleep. Depending
on ability, invite those you care for to find a meaningful breath
prayer and promise to pray it with them. Share your prayer and

ask them to pray it with you. This way of prayer can be a beautiful expression of mutual care.[11]

Scripture Phrase Prayers. A form of prayer many of us do naturally takes short verses of Scripture as a focal point. We each have our favorites:

- "Be still, and know that I am God" (Psalm 46:10).
- "In quietness and trust shall be your strength" (Isaiah 30:15).

Once I realized that Bab's care was my primary spiritual practice, I began drawing on Epistle texts describing the marks of life in Christ and the fruit of the Spirit in us. The following prayers are drawn from Ephesians 4:29–5:2—some in simplified form to make them easier to carry in memory:

- "Put away all bitterness, wrath, and anger."
- "Be kind, tenderhearted, forgiving one another."
- "Live in love, as Christ loved us and gave himself for us."

Here are a few similar phrases from Colossians 3:12–17:

- "Clothe yourself with compassion, kindness, humility, and patience."
- "Bear with one another."
- "Love binds everything together in harmony."
- "Let the peace of Christ rule in your heart."
- "With gratitude, sing hymns and songs to God."

These ways of living were just what I needed in order to offer care faithfully and to be spiritually sustained in my labors. They were also gifts that the Spirit slowly wove into my life through caregiving itself—precisely within all the sacrifice, irritation, discouragement, fatigue, perseverance, and grudging growth!

Henri says something beautiful about how these short phrases work in us. He writes, "When, for instance, we have spent 20 minutes in the early morning sitting in the presence of God with the words, 'The Lord is my shepherd,' they may slowly build a little nest for themselves in our heart and stay there for the rest of our busy day."[12] What a delightful image! We might have only five minutes, but the dynamic is the same. The practice is *not* directed toward deeper insight into God's nature as our shepherd, but toward the *experience* of God's shepherding care in our daily life. Repeating these verses is less an occasion to ponder their meaning than to create inner space for holy Presence—"a little nest in our heart."

5. AFFIRMATIONS

Affirmations have become a familiar practice in recent decades, growing from the self-esteem movement in counseling and therapy. "I'm OK, you're OK" was the famously simplistic cliché of the early movement. An affirmation is a spiritual practice to the degree that it expresses deep confidence in who we are before and in God. In this sense, it resembles a "confession of faith"—not surprisingly also called "an *affirmation* of faith."

The great promises of our faith are ripe with possibility for spiritual affirmations—declared truths that can keep us grounded, hopeful, and steady when life is difficult and the road is long. Perhaps the most sustaining insight Henri came upon was the truth he called "our belovedness." When Henri meditated on the story of Jesus' baptism, he understood that the One who says, "This is my beloved son" speaks the same words to us in *our* baptism. We are each the beloved son or daughter of God. We have been so from long before our birth and will be so long after our death. Here is how Henri once articulated this insight:

Listen to what God is saying to us:
You are my child.
You are written in the palms of my hand.
You are hidden in the shadow of my wing.
I have molded you in the secret of the earth.

I have knitted you together in your mother's womb.

You belong to me.

I am yours. You are mine.

I have called you from eternity and you are the one who is held safe and embraced in love from eternity to eternity.

Whatever happens to you, I am always there. I was always there; I always will be there and hold you in my embrace.

You are my child. You belong to my home. You belong to my intimate life and I will never let you go. I will be faithful to you.[13]

Take a moment to explore the affirmations you could create from this passage. Henri speaks as if with God's voice to us. We can make the phrases ours to speak to God in affirmations of trust and gratitude. A few possibilities:

- I am yours. I belong to your home.
- I am written on the palm of your hand.
- I am safely embraced for all eternity.
- You are faithful and will never let me go.

Such affirmations are a lovely expression of prayer. Rooted in a life-giving word we have heard God speak to us, and directed back to God, they complete the circle of mutual love that is the heart of prayer. Write your affirmations on sticky notes and place them where you will see them daily—atop your dresser, on a mirror, beside your breakfast placemat, or on the edge of your computer. Some people make a running banner of their affirmation, visible as soon as they turn their computer on.

Like breath prayer, the practice of affirmation is wonderful to share with care receivers. Each of you can benefit from your own affirmations, and when you know which ones are meaningful to each other they become another bond between you. You may find yourself reminding the other, when they have forgotten, of their phrase of confident trust or beloved identity.

6. BLESSINGS

When grateful for a happy surprise or thoughtful gesture, we might exclaim, "Oh, bless you!" Apart from that expression, we seem largely to have forgotten how to bless one another in our culture. I have long been moved by the Jewish practice of parents blessing their children at the weekly celebration of Shabbat. What a lovely thing to learn how to bless one another—a God-given power each of us may claim to invoke goodness and grace for others. A blessing conveys not only *our* love but also the unlimited love beneath and beyond our own.

How do we bless each other? A priest or minister offers a "benediction" at the end of worship. Benediction simply means "a good word," and is synonymous with blessing. When we bless each other we say good words: words of gratitude, affirmation, and encouragement; words that draw attention beyond ourselves to the realm of divine presence. The way you express it will be uniquely yours. Perhaps you rest a hand on another's shoulder, or take their hands in yours, meet their eyes, and speak simple, heartfelt words like these:

"You are a great gift to me, and I love you dearly."

"I bless you for your patience with me, and your trust in my care."

"You are so dear to me. May God comfort and fill you with all peace."

"Your inner strength is a witness to me, and I bless you for who you are."

You might instead borrow familiar blessings from Scripture or liturgy that you commit to memory: "The Lord bless you and keep you; the Lord make his face to shine upon you and give you peace." "May God grant you a quiet night and peace at the last." More than a lovely way to say goodnight, such blessings evoke the divine presence we place our trust in both here and beyond this lifetime. For those who know or suspect that they are facing death soon, daily blessings like these can help prepare their spirit for its coming transition to the fullness of God's reign.

You may find that the one you care for would like to bless you in return, confirming a joyful, tender mutuality in your relationship. Receive gratefully!

7. PRACTICING SELF-COMPASSION

As caregivers we often wonder if we are giving all we should, or doing so in the best way. We may carry unrealistic expectations of trying to be perfect. When we feel inadequate or guilty about some failure—real or perceived—it is time for self-compassion.

Self-compassion is a practice of mindfulness. Negative self-talk is the bell calling us to be aware of self-judgment: "I just don't have what it takes to do this." "I was so impatient with him, he must hate me." "Why can't I just say this honestly? I'm such a wimp!" "How could I have forgotten? What an idiot I am!" "God must think I'm a pretty poor specimen." We have choice words for ourselves, and sometimes use them as battering rams.

Can we humbly allow for our human weaknesses? Do we affirm that God loves us even when we are fearful, frustrated, or foolish? Humility and trust are foundations of self-compassion. Think how we look on small children with a knowing tenderness when they inadvertently break a toy or hurt someone without meaning to. Normally we offer comfort and clear but gentle guidance—a pale reflection of God's response when we fail and fall. In his final gesture of forgiveness on the cross, Jesus shows us the unfailing compassion of God not merely for inadvertent but very intentional injuries. From his perspective, we simply don't know what we do. Jesus is God's vulnerable heart revealed.

I love; therefore I am vulnerable.
—MADELEINE L'ENGLE

Since God treats us with compassion, we can offer the same gift to others—and to ourselves. How often we are our own worst critic! When we believe we don't deserve compassion from anyone, especially ourselves, Jesus asks us to be converted to a more generous way—the way of love. We are no more or less deserving of love than anyone else. Thank goodness for "the unflinching father of the prodigal!" It is the freedom and generosity of divine love that allows us to mature and reflect God's love ourselves.

Self-empathy gives us the opportunity to listen to our own hearts with the same quality of compassionate attention that we would offer another in our best moments.
—DEBORAH HUNSINGER

When you are frustrated with yourself, discouraged or dispirited, try out the healing practice called "A Meditation for Compassionate Self-Observation" (see Appendix D).

CONCLUDING THIS STRETCH OF THE JOURNEY

The practices offered here represent a fraction of what is widely available. They are practical ways to help sustain us—body and soul—through the demanding responsibilities of caregiving. We are at liberty to discover what best feeds and replenishes our own spirit for the long haul. Attending to heart and life will provide the best guidance.

Our exploration of the story of caregiving through this book now comes to an end. Our stories will, of course, continue. My fond hope is that you have found helpful ways to name your experience and tell your story; a feeling of being heard in the difficult challenges you face; a greater sense of community with others on this path; new perspectives on your care relationship; self-care and spiritual practices to help sustain you over time; and fresh courage to move forward into God's future with your loved ones, whatever may be the limits of their time or yours on this earth.

Naturally, the final word belongs to love. What else, finally, can we cling to? Is there any higher good, anything beyond the love of God? All our suffering, yearning, sacrifice and service; all our joy, gratitude, and growth toward maturity—it is *all* encompassed by God's love. When our loved ones die, and when we ourselves cross the threshold of death, we will find ourselves fully embraced in the Light that is simply the glorious radiance of divine Love. Even now each of us participates, in our small way, in the Love that will not let us go. Love is the energy and motivation for all care. As we take time to receive that love deeply in our hearts, we have it to give away. What greater privilege and joy can there be? All blessings of grace and peace as you journey forward!

Retreat Leader Guide

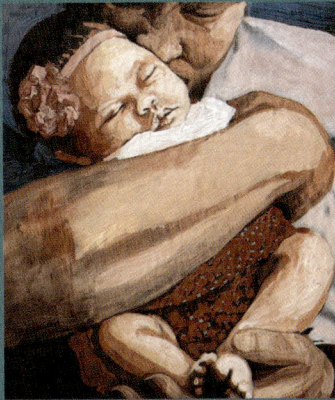

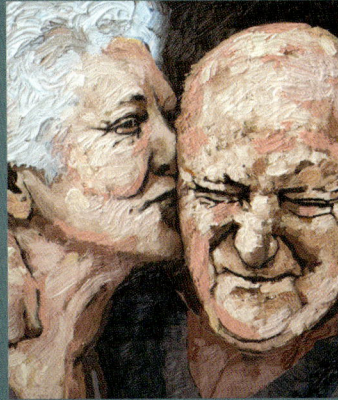

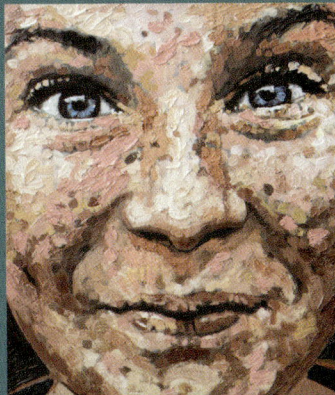

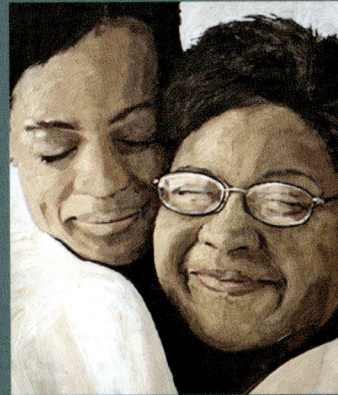

T HE PURPOSE OF THIS Retreat Leader Guide is to help congregational leaders develop one-day retreats for caregivers in their churches and the wider communities they serve. *Courage for Caregivers* is directed to an audience of active caregivers. Persons directly involved in the primary role of daily care responsibilities are unlikely to be able to attend more than a one-day event. What follows is a retreat model limited to a single day and aligned with the companion product, *Courage for Caregivers: A Retreat Participant Workbook* (available separately). So central is the importance of retreat for isolated and overwhelmed caregivers that the participant workbook paired with this guide is written specifically to support this retreat model. The retreat day offers brief opening and closing worship, presented material, periods of personal reflection, and small-group and plenary sharing.

Each participant should have a copy of the Participant Workbook, both for following along with stories, quotations, and content, and for personal reflection on how the wisdom of Henri Nouwen, a few other writers, and the stories of others may help them understand and articulate their own stories more clearly. The workbook will be a record of the retreat experience, but also a physical invitation to continue shaping and sharing those stories. Throughout the day, participants have occasion to reflect personally in spaces labeled "Noting connections to my story ... " You might point this out at the beginning of the day with the assurance that participants may come back to many of these opportunities later for further reflection rather than feel pressure to complete them all during the retreat, when time is limited.

RETREAT LOGISTICS

A smooth and satisfying retreat experience benefits from careful planning. This list covers basic arrangements to plan ahead of time. If possible, find a retreat preparation partner willing to take on details of logistical planning so you can focus on content and process.

Participant Workbook.

All participant materials are incorporated into the Participant Workbook. (If you choose to adapt the time frames from the schedule suggested here, which also appears in the workbook, you will need to create a one-page schedule handout for participants to distribute during registration.)

Centering visual.

Arrange a worship visual at the front of the room near where you will speak. This can be as simple as a small table with a covering cloth, pillar candle, and some symbol (a clear bowl of water with a few smooth stones; a small plant or simple fresh flowers; a cross, icon, or beautiful photograph).

Worship resources.

Arrange for whatever materials or people resources you need for worship. You can easily lead yourself if you wish, or ask others to read a text, lead song, or bring an instrument. If you plan for recorded ambient music, check that all equipment needed is working properly.

Small-group arrangements.

Think through in advance how to structure small groups so that logistics will not take time away from the retreat itself. An easy approach is to put colored sticker dots on name tags and identify groups by sticker color when the time comes. If the setup is at round tables, table groups can comprise small groups. If you know participants in advance, you can group people with similar care situations (elder care, children with disabilities, spousal care). Make sure your meeting space allows small groups not to be too crowded together, or arrange for break-out spaces. With larger groups of eight to ten, it is helpful to have a facilitator in each group who can encourage quieter voices to speak. With groups of four to six, sharing tends to flow well without facilitation.

Sound.

Use a working microphone for the sake of the hearing-impaired.

Lunch.

Arrange lunch so the food can be served on time and within the time frame your schedule allows. You could invite people with similar care circumstances to sit at lunch tables together.

RETREAT SCHEDULE OVERVIEW

8:30   Registration with Coffee, Tea, and Light Snacks

9:00   Welcome, Announcements, and Morning Prayers

9:20   Session 1—The Mutuality of Caregiving:
Henri's Wisdom and Our Stories

     9:20   Part 1: Henri's Wisdom

     9:45   Part 2: Our Stories

10:00   *Break*

10:10   Session 2—The Challenges of Caregiving:
Naming and Embracing

     10:40   Personal Reflection ~ with questions
and journaling

     11:00   Small Groups ~ sharing personal stories,
connections, questions

     11:40   Plenary ~ gathering insights and questions

12:00   *Lunch*

1:00   Session 3—The Gifts of Caregiving:
Seeing and Celebrating

     1:30   Personal Reflection ~ with questions
or writing a letter

     1:50   Small Groups ~ sharing personal experience

2:30   *Break*

2:40   Session 4—The Sustenance of Caregiving:
Self-care and Spiritual Practice

     3:20   Plenary ~ gathering insights and
sharing resources

3:45   Evening Prayers

4:00   *Goodbyes*

Courage for Caregivers Retreat:
Expanded Outline for Leader

9:00 — ### WELCOME AND ANNOUNCEMENTS

Make the welcome warm and keep logistical announcements to a minimum. Be sure to draw attention to the retreat schedule in the *Courage for Caregivers: A Retreat Participant Workbook* (page 7). Assure participants that all sharing is at one's personal discretion. Whether in small groups or plenary, share as you are comfortable.

9:05 — ### MORNING PRAYERS

For Morning and Evening Prayers, see Appendix D (page 141). Brief times of worship bookend the retreat. Invite a quiet seeking of God's presence along with Scripture, prayer, and song. This time needs to offer breathing space for people who come to the retreat "out of breath." Worship times serve to help participants decompress, settle, and become more fully present. While relatively short, they should not feel rushed.

9:20 — ### SESSION 1
The Mutuality of Caregiving:
Henri's Wisdom and Our Stories

This content segment is carefully crafted and paced. It incorporates material from two portions of this book, Beginnings: Henri Nouwen, Our Spiritual Companion and Chapter 1, The Mutuality of Caregiving: Shared Suffering and Compassion, but not necessarily in the order you find the material there. The goal is two-fold:

1. To ground our consideration of caregiving in Henri's wisdom.
2. To begin thinking of our own caregiving experience as a story.

PART 1: HENRI'S WISDOM (20–25 MINUTES).

Sketch keys to Henri's wisdom on care by highlighting the following:

1. Henri Nouwen's wisdom will be a source of guidance through the day. Some quotes will be read aloud to consider as a group. Others may not be used in group discussion but are available for participants to reflect on personally. As you lead the group through the workbook, assure them that while not everything in it will be mentioned during the retreat day, it will be valuable to reflect on and write personal responses to as they continue to process their own caregiving stories beyond this retreat.

   Begin by inviting someone to read aloud the paragraph on Henri's life in relation to caring under *Henri Nouwen—Our Spiritual Companion* (Participant Workbook, page 10).

2. Draw from *Caregiving: Universal and Unique*, paragraph 1 (*Courage for Caregivers, Beginnings*, page 16).

   The routines and responsibilities of caregiving can leave us feeling deeply isolated. Yet we are not alone; caring is a universal experience. Henri writes, "To care is the most human of all gestures." And, "Caring is the privilege of every person and is at the heart of being human." We are in this adventure of faithful caregiving together.

3. Articulate the Three Keys to Henri's perspective on care.
   - Care is not cure: true care allows us to be comfortable with weakness.
   - Care expresses and expands our compassion, understood as suffering with others.
   - Care draws us into profound mutuality, both in shared vulnerability and shared gifts.

4. Describe briefly Henri's distinction between care and cure:
   Care professionals are often so focused on *cure* that real *care*

is neglected and patients may feel depersonalized. In contrast, Henri describes the value of authentic care. Invite another participant to read the quote that begins, "What is care? … " (Participant Workbook, page 12).

5. Draw out Henri's teaching on compassion—ours and God's.
   - The word compassion comes from the Latin *pati* (to bear or suffer) and *cum* (with). Compassion means "to bear with" or "suffer with." It is the *ability to feel with the other.*
   - Our hearts have a strong impulse to feel with others, yet we have an equally powerful resistance to feeling too much! Invite a participant to read Henri's quote: "Compassion is hard because … " (Participant Workbook, page 13).
   - Henri notes that God joins us precisely in the difficulty we have facing our suffering. Ask someone to read the quote, "There can be no human beings … " (page 14).

6. While suffering is unavoidable on both sides of the care relationship, pain is not the final word.
   - Blessings and joys are part of the experience as well. So we divide our retreat day into a morning session on naming *challenges* of our care experience, and an afternoon session lifting up the *gifts* of caregiving.
   - Henri gets at joyful aspects of caring in his teaching on the *deep mutuality at the heart of every care relationship.* Invite another voice to read Henri's quote: "In the very act of caring … " (Participant Workbook, page 15).
   - Read the story of Henri's learning with Adam (Chapter 1, under "Care and the Treasure of Mutuality"), beginning with "Henri illustrates …" through the quote on Adam as his teacher (page 26).
   - Invite another voice to read the quote beginning, "Those who ask for care … " (Participant Workbook, page 17). Remind participants that this retreat is a good opportunity for each

of us to consider how mutuality is present in our own experience of caregiving. If you have a few minutes to spare, give participants an opportunity to jot a few connections to their personal stories in the workbook writing space after this quote.

PART 2: OUR STORIES (15 MINUTES).

Introduce people to "Our Stories." Tie this in with the end of the segment on Henri above by explaining that this retreat also gives us an opportunity to think about our caregiving experience *as a story*, something we may not have fully considered. We will have time to begin that process by responding to a few questions before the break. But first take 10 minutes to look at the theme of story more generally.

1. Turn together in the workbook to page 17, and invite someone to read the paragraph under "Our Storied Lives," beginning with, "Stories are essential ... "

2. Explain that you will be working with several stories from the materials through the day, but stress that the group's own stories are equally important. Condense in your own words the essence of the second paragraph under the heading "Our Storied Lives" on page 15 in Beginnings.

3. Briefly acknowledge the variety of care circumstances and settings we can find ourselves in, naming a few examples from the next section in Beginnings, "Caregiving: Universal and Unique," (page 16). Explain that while those gathered for the retreat have different personal situations, in sharing varied stories participants can find common ground and expand their understanding.

4. Invite people to look at the workbook under "Your Caregiving Story" (page 18) and begin to think about the broad contours of their own care stories by responding briefly to the questions

there. They have only five minutes for this exercise; it's just a start.

10:00 — *BREAK*

10:10 — # SESSION 2
The Challenges of Caregiving: Naming and Embracing

The next half hour is your opportunity to invite retreat participants to tell stories about the challenges of both giving and receiving care. As author, I have shared my own stories more fully than others. If you have direct caregiving experience, it may be more effective to tell something of your story and supplement it with selected portions of Chapter 2, The Challenges of Caregiving: Naming and Embracing.

Turn together to page 22 in the workbook and point out Henri's perspective in the quote that appears in the introductory paragraph at the start of Session 2.

TAILOR THE PRESENTATION TO YOUR GROUP.
Here are several general categories and a few specific elements that are important to include.

1. Look over the common challenges listed in the workbook (page 23) for five general categories to incorporate into your stories or to identify in the caregiving story of another person you choose to use. You need not illustrate every possibility identified *within* those categories. These five categories correlate with some of the questions participants will respond to in their personal reflection time.

2. Try to touch on the following elements from Chapter 2.
   • *The importance of honestly naming hard experiences and feelings* (page 41). Only when we allow, acknowledge, own, and honor our real feelings can we fully accept them. As feelings become more integrated into our conscious lives,

we can move toward healing and transformation. Speaking the hard realities aloud may also help us see where we need support.

• *The cumulative impact of caregiving over the long haul,* especially if care receiver needs increase with time (pages 42–43). You could illustrate this diagram on a chart with the vertical dimension representing your energy level and the horizontal dimension representing your care receiver's needs over time. Your line will start high and slowly drop over time, while the needs line starts low and moves higher; eventually the two lines cross and the needs become higher than your energy to meet them.

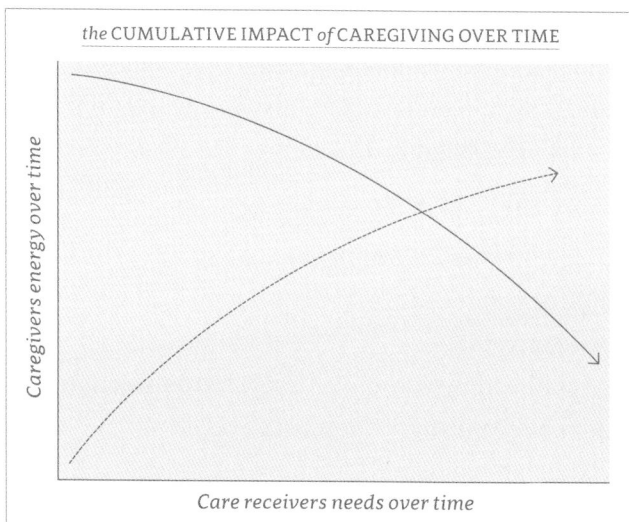

the CUMULATIVE IMPACT *of* CAREGIVING OVER TIME

Caregivers energy over time

Care receivers needs over time

• *The interruption of caregiving in our lives and the expectations we hold around our sense of purpose or vocation* (pages 43–44). What might it mean to fully embrace or freely choose a life that feels "unchosen?" (This points us toward spiritual practices to be addressed more fully in the final session this afternoon.)

3. Leave the final five to eight minutes of your presentation for a short segment on *challenges for care receivers*. You might invite a participant to read Henri's quote on page 32 of the workbook and add comments based on your own experience, or you could draw an illustration from the end of Chapter 2.

10:40

MORNING PERSONAL REFLECTION ACTIVITY.

Invite participants to turn to page 34 in the workbook, where they will find reflection questions based on this session. The next 20 minutes are a gift of personal quiet time to reflect on questions that call out to them and journal their responses in the blank pages provided. Instruct the group to honor this period of silence. They may quietly attend to restroom or refreshment needs. Depending on room size and weather, you could encourage them to stay in their seats or find their own spaces in the room or outside. Be sure you have an audible way to call people back if they are leaving the room. (A bell or chime works well.)

11:00

SMALL GROUPS.

Indicate that this is an opportunity for the groups to share whatever personal reflections they wish to. Some questions that might spur conversation:

- What connections have you discovered between the morning content and our own stories of caregiving?
- What insights or questions have emerged?

11:40

PLENARY SHARING.

Spend a little time before the lunch break inviting sharing within the large group. Gather up diverse experiences for all to hear. What insights or connections are arising at the individual and small-group levels? Encourage people to use lunch conversation for further sharing. Point out "Questions to Carry into My Life from the Morning Session" (page 36 in the workbook), which participants may want to reflect on when they are home in their own settings. Then draw attention to the shift that happens after lunch, when the discussion will turn from the challenges of caregiving to its gifts.

LUNCH — 12:00

SESSION 3
The Gifts of Caregiving: Seeing and Celebrating

— 1:00

Look through the Participant Workbook for this session so you can work in tandem with the portions of text participants are seeing.

GROUP OVERVIEW (30 MINUTES).

1. In the first five minutes:

    • Make the turn from challenges, explored in Session 2, to gifts, briefly naming the truth that care relationships bring *mutual blessing* as well as struggle.

    • Give everyone two minutes to read silently the three paragraphs introducing this session on page 40 in the workbook, underlining phrases that stand out to them.

    • Then invite them to share one phrase aloud, "popcorn style" around the room, without comment or discussion.

2. Take the next 20 minutes to share stories about the gifts caregivers discover in the midst of caregiving. Feel free to draw on your own experience along with stories from Chapter 3, The Gifts of Caregiving: Seeing and Celebrating. Portions of two "Stories of Gift" from this chapter appear in the workbook, A Story with Jean and A Story with Bab. One approach: Ask varied voices from the group to read a paragraph each of one story, followed by three or four minutes for journaling in the space provided. You could use this pattern with both stories, and still have some time to add perspectives of your own.

3. Leave the last five minutes to touch on "Gifts from Our Care Receivers."
   - Ask someone to read the quote from Henri on page 46 in the workbook that begins, "The bodily resurrection ... "
   - Illustrate this wisdom with the words of Donna, mother of the high-needs child named Nicholas. Read from Chapter 3, page 65, beginning with "We *want* to give care" through "it is so deeply satisfying."

1:30   AFTERNOON REFLECTION ACTIVITY OPTIONS.

Explain that participants will have 20 minutes for personal reflection and may use the time one of two ways.

1. The first option is journal responses to the personal reflection questions found on page 49 of the workbook.

2. The second option is to write a letter of appreciation to a loved one for the blessings received in caring for him or her. The workbook also includes space for doing this (page 52).

1:50   SMALL GROUPS.

Call everyone back from individual reflection time. Encourage participants to gather in their small groups and share briefly their insights from personal reflection or letter writing.

2:30   *BREAK*

2:40   SESSION 4

The Sustenance of Caregiving:
Self-care and Spiritual Practice

You have 40 minutes to cover two distinct but related areas: 20 minutes for Self-care and another 20 minutes for Spiritual Practice. Be familiar with the Participant Workbook and select carefully how to focus each area. Here is one way to proceed, but you may adapt according to your sense of the needs of your group.

SELF-CARE.

Turn together in the workbook to page 56 and ask for two voices to read the opening paragraphs aloud. Then proceed with these steps, moving back and forth between presenting material and allowing time for participants to record or share their own responses.

1. Self-care is a tender topic for caregivers. Lindsey acknowledges, "It's so hard to hear, 'Take care of yourself.' It's like someone telling a person who is already completely overwhelmed that there's one more thing they need to do!" The message often comes from close family members or friends who are not in a position to help. They are expressing fear for her well-being, and that fear becomes one more weight for Lindsey to carry. Donna says that self-care advice from others, however well-meant, often "just feels like an exercise in shaming"—especially when given instead of real support or practical help. Nonetheless, Lindsey and Donna well know that self-care is critical to survival when you live in the trenches of long-term caregiving!

2. Allow a few minutes for people to reflect on the first two questions on page 58 about how they respond to the topic of self-care: What feelings arise when others urge me to "take care of myself"? and What makes self-care most difficult for me?

3. Under the heading "Self-care Practices" in the workbook, ask a participant to read the quote by Michelle O'Rourke and the paragraph following, where Donna challenges caregivers to a new way of imagining self-nurture.
   - Give a few minutes for people to reflect and journal on the set of questions following Donna's challenge.
   - Then read the paragraph beginning "Donna suggests … "

Invite people to return later to the questions listed after this paragraph for reflection on their own time.

- Palliative care nurse Michelle O'Rourke's asks two questions. Point these out, and have various voices read aloud one line each of the self-care suggestions on page 62.

Before leaving the topic of self-care, underscore the point about boundaries opening up space and Henri's advice for avoiding burnout as a caregiver.

REALISTIC SPIRITUAL PRACTICES.
In this limited time, you can only indicate a few points about these practices and perhaps offer a brief taste of one. Point out that fairly complete descriptions of each practice are included in the Participant Workbook because these are important resources for participants to return to at home for spiritual sustenance. If you have time for a five-minute exercise, invite people to write a few stanzas of their own psalm of lament or to create a Breath Prayer for themselves.

Here is a way to proceed:
Invite someone to read the opening paragraph in the Participant Workbook on page 64 under the heading Realistic Spiritual Practices. Then make these points in an overview of the practices. All page numbers below reference the workbook.

Honest lament.
Point to Praying the Psalms (page 65) and encourage this practice. Have someone read the sample paraphrase.

Reframing.
- Briefly describe reframing, based on the opening paragraph of page 66.
- Point out two short illustrations of reframing, based on the stories you have chosen to share or those printed in the workbook.

Say a word about Jesus' way of reframing life from a "kingdom perspective."

Holy Listening.

- Name a few ways of listening to ourselves.
- Read Donna's description of listening to Nicholas to illustrate hearing others "speak" beyond words. (See Chapter 4, page 82.)

Simple Prayers.

- In pointing briefly to the workbook examples of Breath Prayer and Scripture Phrase prayer, ask if some of the group already use such prayers naturally.
- Underscore how practical these prayers are for busy caregivers, and how helpful they can be to care receivers as well.

Affirmations.

- Indicate that while these are similar to single-phrase prayers, they are more like affirmations of faith and trust. Participants can read about these later and create their own.

Blessings.

- Underscore how valuable it can be in care relationships to bless one another. Invite participants to look briefly at the bulleted list on page 72.
- Mention the value of scriptural blessings associated with evening prayers for people who face death in the near term (the metaphor of "the evening of life" is deeply embedded in Christian consciousness).

Self-compassion.

- Last but not least, when we suffer from self-recrimination and perfectionism the practice of self-compassion is deeply important for caregivers!
- Invite someone to read the quote on self-empathy.
- Indicate that the "Meditation for Compassionate Self-observation"

is a helpful practice to learn, and encourage participants to try it out on their own.

If you have time, give everyone five minutes to write a few stanzas of their own psalm of lament, or to find a Breath Prayer or Scripture phrase they wish to live with awhile.

3:30 — PLENARY SHARING.

In this final opportunity to debrief together, offer space for participants to reflect on the insights from the day that have been most significant to them personally. Here are some questions that might help people focus their thought on what they will take away from the day.

- What has been most surprising or meaningful to you about this day?
- Where have conversations taken you today that you didn't expect to go?
- What themes or practices from today do you hope to revisit in the days ahead?
- How would you tell your story of being a caregiver differently as a result of participating in the *Courage for Caregivers* retreat?

Appendix D contains assorted resources that can be distributed as handouts for participants to use for further reading and meditation. These are not required. You may select some to prepare as packets, or you might prefer to make them available on a resource table and let individuals pick up the ones they are interested in. The end of this plenary sharing is a good time to point out that these are available.

3:45 — EVENING PRAYERS

4:00 — *GOODBYES*

Small Group Leader Guide

For Home Groups, Adult Classes, Support Groups, Congregational Care Teams, Health Ministry Teams, and Workshops

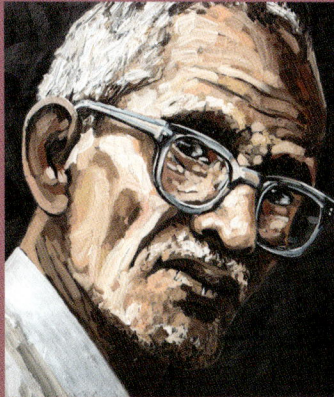

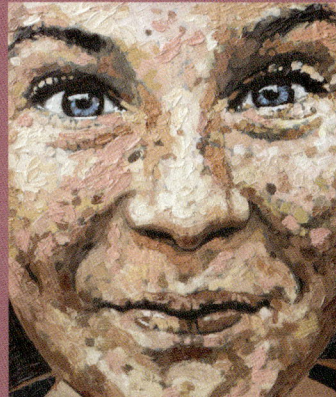

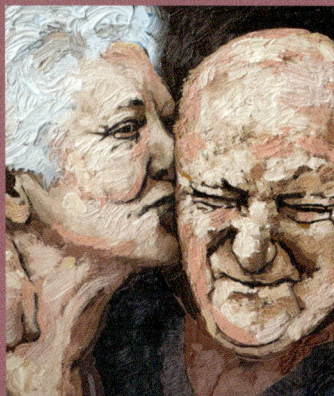

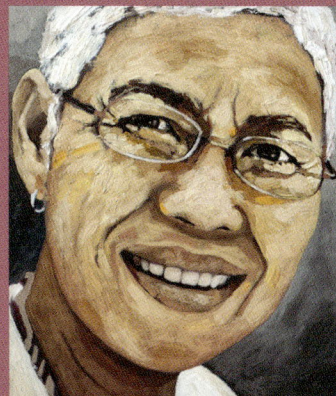

C OURAGE FOR CAREGIVERS is a flexible resource appropriate for use with small groups within a congregation that wish to explore the topic of caregiving. This may be in adult Sunday school class settings, small groups meeting in homes, a series of meetings for members of a congregational care ministry team or health teams, or a one-day workshop and discussion event that includes both people in caregiving roles and others learning more about the topic.

Why use *Courage for Caregivers* in small groups? Here are three ways that your small group or congregation can benefit.

1. *Acknowledge the growing need.* Caregiving is a universal experience. Henri Nouwen said that "caring is the privilege of every person and is at the heart of being human." Some of us find ourselves in more demanding caregiving situations than we expected, whether in caring for children with special needs, family members with unexpected illness or disability, or aging parents. In particular, as people live longer, care for aging adults is a growing need.

2. *Increase awareness and conversation.* Not everyone cares for a child with intense needs or an aging parent, but virtually everyone knows someone who does. Reading and discussing the concepts and stories of *Courage for Caregivers* opens a window into what life is like for caregivers, which in turn opens channels of empathy and understanding.

3. *Develop congregational support.* Empathy and understanding will lead to practical congregational support for members of the faith community whose lives are consumed with caregiving. Small groups discussing *Courage for Caregivers* can help people find points of identification with caregiving and lay a foundation to care for the caregivers.

The material that follows in this guide suggests a structure for four one-hour sessions based on the four chapters of *Courage for Caregivers*. Participants in these sessions should be encouraged to obtain a copy of the book and read in advance the chapter that will be discussed in each session. If your group has more time, or is interested to dig deeper into discussion, you may choose to divide the material and expand the number of sessions. Always be sure to invite group members to share their own caregiving stories and experiences as they relate to the topic of each session.

The structure is simple.

- READ aloud select passages from each chapter.

- RESPOND to suggested prompts by leading a simple discussion that invites everyone to participate.

- REVIEW some basic content from the chapter. Brief summaries are provided, but you may augment them with further content from the chapter that you consider relevant to your group or setting. Be sure to encourage group members to share points from the chapters that most resonate with them.

- REFLECT on personal connections.

This structure repeats as the group works through each section of the chapter.

SESSION 1

The Mutuality of Caregiving:
Shared Suffering and Compassion

Welcome everyone to the first session of Courage for Caregivers. Affirm that the purpose of these sessions is to gain a deeper understanding of what we give and receive in caregiving as we learn from the wisdom of Henri Nouwen and reflect on our own experiences of caregiving.

Henri's Wisdom on Care versus Cure

READ

Ask someone to turn to page 20 and read the opening paragraph identifying three key insights about care.

RESPOND

- Which of these three insights resonates with you most immediately? Why?

REVIEW

Care professionals are often so focused on *cure* that real *care* is neglected and patients may feel depersonalized. In contrast, Henri describes the value of authentic care, reminding us that to care is to "cry out with those who are ill, confused, lonely, isolated, and forgotten, and to recognize their pains with our own heart." To care is to be present and remain present even when we cannot change the situation, when we cannot alter the circumstances.

REFLECT

- Think about a situation in which you wished you could change the situation for the better but could not. Were you able to recognize that even though you couldn't change things, authentic care was still possible? If so, what was that realization like for you?

- What factors in our culture and in ourselves make it difficult for us to live comfortably with the distinction between cure and care?

Suffering and Compassion

READ

Turn to page 23 and ask someone to read aloud the two paragraphs beginning with "How many are the ways we recoil from physical and mental anguish!"

RESPOND

- Henri acknowledged that the question "Why?" spontaneously emerges in the face of suffering. What role has your faith story played in helping you cope with this question?

REVIEW

Henri understood how faith sustains and strengthens us in our suffering, even when the questions are hard. God came to us in Jesus not to take our pains away but to share them with us. God became a part of our suffering. All human suffering is held in God's heart and embraced by divine love. Jesus assures us that he will be with us in our suffering. Because of God's love, no one needs to be alone in suffering. God, in and through Jesus, has become Emmanuel, God with us. The apostle Paul assures us that as we die with Christ, so we shall enter into his resurrected life. These are all powerful promises to hold—and allow to hold us—when we are grieved by the sufferings of those we care for, and worn down by the relentlessness of giving care.

REFLECT

- Read Philippians 2:5–8. What do these verses tell us about the way God enters our suffering?
- Jesus said "yes" to a cup of suffering and sorrow. Our culture often wants us to believe that the perfect life would be free of suffering. How can followers of Jesus hold—and speak—a

different understanding of suffering?

- As we engage our suffering and that of others with courage, we discover growing compassion. How have you experienced the relationship between suffering and compassion?

Care and the Treasure of Mutuality

READ

Turn to page 25 and ask someone to read the opening paragraph, beginning with, "While care involves us unavoidably in suffering, it would be a great mistake ... "

RESPOND

- Why do we most often think of the suffering side of care first before considering the treasure of mutuality?

REVIEW

During the years Henri lived in the L'Arche Community of Daybreak, he cared for Adam, a severely disabled man who could not walk, speak, or care for his needs in any way. Henri discovered that Adam had his own way of communicating and was capable of offering a profound sense of presence. In fact, Henri found himself confiding in Adam and felt that Adam was listening with his whole being. He went so far as to say that Adam became his teacher, walking with him through the wilderness of his life. Henri's inner handicaps may have been less visible than Adam's disabilities, but they were just as real. Henri helps us to see our shared human vulnerability as a source of belonging, comfort, and community. We are "wounded healers" for each other. By acknowledging our own wounds, we can bring an authentic healing presence to others in pain.

REFLECT

- Henri discovered a mutuality of caregiving in his relationship with Adam because he was able to move beyond conventional ideas of who was caring for whom. They cared for each other in different ways. What valuable treasures might await us in caregiving if we are able to open ourselves up beyond the roles we expect?

- Share an experience where you have realized your own vulnerability and offered it to another person. In what way did the experience illustrate Henri's concept of being "wounded healers"?

Close the session with a time of prayer. If your group is accustomed to sharing personal requests, use this time as you normally do. Some of the reflection questions may have revealed stories that would be appropriate to support with prayer at this time as well. If your group is accustomed to closing by having one person pray, gather thanks and praise for the insights and blessings of your time together.

SESSION 2
The Challenges of Caregiving: Naming and Embracing

Welcome everyone to the second session of Courage for Caregivers. Take a couple of quick moments to invite reflection on the first session in the days since you last met.

Challenges for the Caregiver
READ

Remind the group that the second chapter includes narratives of the author's experiences of being a primary caregiver for both her mother and her mother-in-law that capture many common challenges caregivers in the group may easily identify with—and non-caregivers can learn from. Turn to page 30 and ask someone to read the first paragraph to introduce the chapter.

RESPOND

- What emotions do you feel at encountering the topic of "challenges" for the caregiver?

REVIEW

Ask group members to turn to page 30 to remind themselves of the author's accounts of the challenges of caring for Jean and Bab. If time permits, select a few paragraphs to read aloud that highlight the challenges identified. These include: balancing the needs of the caregiver and the care receiver; getting adequate rest; attending to *needs* and to *desires* with limited time and energy; physical stress; conflicting emotions. Other stories in the chapter, from Lindsey and Karen, give raw pictures of the constancy of care for children with severe disability. They indicate the stresses—or even dissolution—of marriage as a cost of intensive caregiving. Point out that Appendix C, A Treasury of Stories, offers additional pictures of the challenges of caregiving that group members may want to read on their own.

Only when we allow, acknowledge, own, and honor our real feelings can we fully accept them. As feelings become more integrated into our conscious lives, we can move toward healing and transformation. Speaking the hard realities aloud may also help us see where we need support. Caregiving has a cumulative impact over the long haul, especially if the care receiver's needs increase with time. Also, the intrusion of caregiving into our lives and the interruption of expectations we hold around our sense of purpose and vocation may be a difficult adjustment.

REFLECT

- Turn to page 41 and review the range of emotions (in the italicized words) that come with caregiving. Why do we sometimes avoid naming the hard things honestly?
- What might it mean to fully embrace and freely choose a caregiving life that feels "unchosen"?
- What new perspective has reflecting on the challenges for the caregiver given you?

Challenges for the Care Receiver

READ

Turn to page 45 and ask someone to read aloud the quote from Henri that begins, "Important for us as caregivers to remember ... "

RESPOND

- What experiences have you had that could help you perceive the care experience from the perspective of the care receiver?

REVIEW

For people who have lived an independent life, letting go of self-sufficiency and accepting help from others is a difficult stage of life. Whether this transition comes through age, illness, or injury, it brings with it a profound sense of loss. The feeling of loss takes many forms—loss of "how things were," loss of control over your body, your personal environment, or decisions that affect you. Such changes and limitations are hard to accept. In addition, it is painful to feel like a burden to those who must now rearrange their lives to provide care for you. The caregiving relationship at all stages of life remains a relationship of respect between full human beings.

REFLECT

- Next time you are in a situation of offering care, even briefly, how might you think differently about the interaction from the perspective of the person receiving your care?
- What safeguards can caregivers take to ensure that they recognize and respect the challenges that care receivers experience?

Close the session with a time of prayer. If your group is accustomed to sharing personal requests, use this time as you normally do. Some of the reflection questions may have revealed stories that would be appropriate to support with prayer at this time as well.

If your group is accustomed to closing by having one person pray, gather thanks and praise for the insights and blessings of your time together.

SESSION 3
The Gifts of Caregiving: Seeing and Celebrating

Welcome everyone to Session 3 of Courage for Caregivers. Take a few minutes to invite insights group members may have had in the days since you were last together.

Our Belovedness: The Ground of Gifts
READ

Turn to page 52 and ask someone to read aloud the first paragraph under the heading "Our Belovedness: The Ground of Gifts."

RESPOND

• How does a sense of belonging to a God who loves us unconditionally affect our perspectives on caregiving?

REVIEW

Henri Nouwen never ceased to proclaim that we are all beloved children of God. Caregivers are called to recognize that the person receiving care is as dearly loved by God as we—even if that person is the crabbiest curmudgeon on the planet; even if that person lies on a bed in an unresponsive state day upon day; even if that person's behavior is difficult to understand or tolerate. These beloved ones of God are truly our teachers if we allow them to be—as many caregivers have discovered with time. Henri delighted to begin his talks with the theme of our belovedness. He would say, in essence, "Listen deeply to the voice of the great lover of souls. Hear that you are beloved. Then you can see that others are, too."

REFLECT

• Share about a time you listened deeply to the great lover of souls and knew your own belovedness—at least for that moment. The gift may have come through Scripture, prayer, nature, or another person who echoed God's love to you.

- What gets in the way of seeing the belovedness in other people? What actions or attitudes might we cultivate so that we see their belovedness more clearly?

Recognizing the Gifts of Caregiving

READ

Turn to page 54 and ask someone to read aloud the two paragraphs that begin, "I can identify several particular gifts we enjoyed ... ," which continue the story of Jean. Then turn to page 58 and read the two paragraphs that begin, "Accompanying our loved ones through caregiving ... ," which continue the story of Bab.

RESPOND

- The challenges of caregiving are easy to see. In what ways do we have to look a little deeper to see the gifts of caregiving?

REVIEW

It is a spiritual challenge to "see Christ in his distressing guise" (a favorite phrase of Mother Teresa of Calcutta). Yet Jesus teaches unequivocally: "I was sick and you took care of me;" and "just as you did it for one of the least of these ... you did it for me" (Matthew 25:36, 40). It takes a faithful imagination to see the image of God in every person. There are times—unexpected moments breaking through the crust of ordinary perception—when God gives us eyes to see the hidden Christ in broken and beloved humanity. What could be more precious than to see the face of our humble Lord shining in the flesh and bone of another human being, weak and imperfect as we all are? What better gift could there be in this world?

REFLECT

- If you have been a caregiver, even for a short season, what gifts have you experienced in that role? If your observations have been more secondhand, share what has inspired you in the caregiving you have witnessed.

- Every caregiving circumstance is its own story. Even if we are not active in caregiving roles, how can we be aware of the realities, needs, and gifts of caregivers by learning their stories?

More Stories of Gift

READ

Turn to page 60 and ask someone to read aloud Lindsey's description of the gifts of caregiving, which begins with, "Who nurtures who more?" Then skip down to Karen's description, which begins with, "I had this little person in my life … " Both paragraphs continue stories introduced in the previous chapter.

RESPOND

- What surprises you most about the way Lindsey and Karen express the gifts of caregiving in the extreme circumstances of their lives?

REVIEW

There is so much in life that we don't sign on for. Yet the most stringent struggles may bring the most light. Karen and Lindsey know by experience that as we allow ourselves to grow through the immense challenges put before us, they bring with them a much richer life experience. They would understand Henri perfectly when he writes in *The Return of the Prodigal Son*, "People who have come to know the joy of God do not deny the darkness, but they choose not to live in it. They claim that the light that shines in the darkness can be trusted more than the darkness itself and that a little bit of light can dispel a lot of darkness." The challenges of life can strengthen as well as weaken our closest relationships. Much depends on our choices and in a marriage, those choices must be held by both partners.

REFLECT

- What tends to be your instinctive response to situations in your life that turned out not to be what you signed on for? If your instinct is negative, how do you get past it?
- In what experiences have you chosen *not* to live in the darkness but rather claim that the light can be trusted more?

Gifts from the Perspectives of Care Receivers

READ

Turn to page 64 and read aloud the first three paragraphs, which continue the stories of Jean and Bab and give us a piece of Henri's wisdom.

RESPOND

- How do you respond to the idea that our weakness can bear fruit in the lives of others?

REVIEW

Henri knew Jesus as the wounded, compassionate One, knowing anguish and anger, knowing how these can be transfigured by grace to genuine blessedness. The father of the Prodigal Son was Henri's central image of the tender, persevering love of God—for himself and for us all. Moreover, Henri saw that once this love is deeply received, it is what we are called to embody. He wrote in *The Return of the Prodigal Son*, "What I do know with unwavering certainty is the heart of the father. It is a heart of limitless mercy … I now see that the hands that forgive, console, heal, and offer a festive meal must become my own."

REFLECT

- In what ways does the image of the father in the story of the Prodigal Son (Luke 15:11–32) speak to you?
- We started this session talking about belovedness. In what ways does the image of the Prodigal Son, who received such lavish love, speak to you?

Close the session with a time of prayer. If your group is accustomed to sharing personal requests, use this time as you normally do. Some of the reflection questions may have revealed stories that would be appropriate to support with prayer at this time as well. If your group is accustomed to closing by having one person pray, gather thanks and praise for the insights and blessings of your time together.

SESSION 4
The Sustenance of Caregiving:
Self-care and Spiritual Practice
Welcome group members to Session 4 of Courage for Caregivers and invite brief reflections on the material you've been studying since the last time you were together.

The Tensions of Sustainable Care
READ
In this session, the discussion turns to care for the caregiver. Turn to page 70 and read aloud the opening two paragraphs beginning with, "Caregiving is a complex mix ... "

RESPOND
- What do you think are some of the biggest challenges for caregivers in taking care of themselves while they have primary responsibility for the care of someone else?

REVIEW
For centuries, Western culture has burdened us with the notion that caring for ourselves is somehow selfish. When we are exhausted, the care we offer others suffers as well. And God does not require us to ruin our health to prove our love! Jesus models balance when he withdraws from the crowds to take time apart for prayer and inner renewal. Yet self-care is a tender topic for caregivers. Often the advice for caregivers to take care of themselves comes in lieu of practical support. And self-care *is* important

for caregivers who face years of intensive caregiving. When we are in the trenches of long-term or sustained intensive care of others, self-care of some kind is not simply optional.

REFLECT

- Why do you think our culture places so little value on self-care?
- What are some important ways we can support caregivers beyond just saying, "Take care of yourself"?

Broad Self-care Practices

READ

Turn to page 71 and read the first two paragraphs under the heading "Broad Self-care Practices." The first shares advices from a palliative care nurse, and the second shows how this advice can be used in the life of a caregiver. Then ask someone to read the list of self-care suggestions bulleted on pages 73–74.

RESPOND

- If you were to be intentional about changing one or two things in your daily routines for better self-care, what would they be?

REVIEW

Shifts in awareness lead to shifts in behavior that result in better self-care. Reframing simple acts can move us toward a more conscious sense of mutuality, along with greater ease and enjoyment in the care relationship. Making our needs known to others, even the person receiving our care, deepens mutuality and strengthens the capacity of everyone in the family to be thoughtful. We will not be able to exercise every self-care strategy every day, but if we are aware of our needs and intentionally tend to them more frequently, self-care practices will bring balance and renewal that is critical for caregivers. There may be some care tasks and responsibilities that we choose to hang onto, but there likely are others that we would be happy to delegate if we had the opportunity. This is another area in which to cultivate awareness and intentionality. We are created for community, to bear one another's burdens and so fulfill the law of Christ (Galatians 6:2).

REFLECT

- What is your own experience with self-care? Does it tend to be at the bottom of your list, or do you have intentional habits?
- Think further about Galatians 6:2 and how being in community with others relates to self-care. What principles might we draw out, both in giving and receiving care?

Realistic Spiritual Practices

READ

Turn to page 76 and read the first two introductory paragraphs under this heading.

RESPOND

- In what ways have you struggled with spiritual practices in your life? In what ways have you found spiritual practices enriching?

REVIEW

The seven spiritual practices for caregivers presented in Chapter 4 are:

1. *Honest lament.* Scripture gives us permission to express the full range of human emotions. We see this in the book of Job and perhaps most fully in the Psalms, where praise and grief, joy and sorrow, contentment and fury contend with each other on every page—sometimes in the same psalm!

2. *Reframing.* We are largely unaware of deeply held assumptions and the interpretations that follow them. Gaining new perspective can give us a different frame of reference, and thus a new story line.

3. *Holy listening.* Listening becomes a spiritual practice when we discover it as sacred ground. Caregiving is a tremendous opportunity to learn how to listen more deeply to ourselves, to others, and to God.

4. *Simple prayer.* What makes listening a holy act is recognizing divine presence at the heart of everything—whether in hearing our inner world more clearly, or in listening openly to another, or in turning our attention directly to the Holy One. Listening to God in the midst of daily challenge and gift is the crux of prayer.

5. *Affirmations.* The great promises of our faith are ripe with possibility for spiritual affirmations—declared truths that can keep us grounded, hopeful, and steady when life is difficult and the road is long.

6. *Blessings.* What a lovely thing to learn how to bless one another—a God-given power each of us may claim to invoke goodness and grace for others. A blessing conveys not only *our* love, but the unlimited love beneath and beyond our own.

7. *Practicing self-compassion.* Can we humbly allow for our human weaknesses? Do we affirm that God loves us even when we are fearful, frustrated, or foolish? Humility and trust are foundations of self-compassion.

REFLECT

- Which of these practices seems to draw you in more naturally?
- Which practices are less familiar but intriguing enough that you might want to explore them further?
- If you are not in the role of being a primary caregiver, which of these might help you to connect with and support a caregiver?

Close the session with a time of prayer. If your group is accustomed to sharing personal requests, use this time as you normally do. Some of the reflection questions may have revealed stories that would be appropriate to support with prayer at this time as well. If your group is accustomed to closing by having one person pray, gather thanks and praise for the insights and blessings of your time together.

A Treasury of Stories

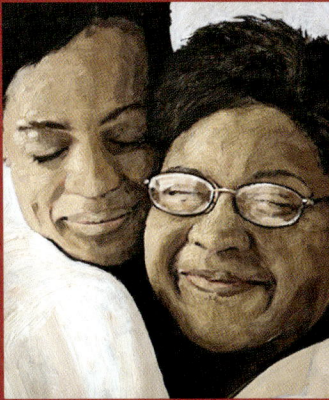

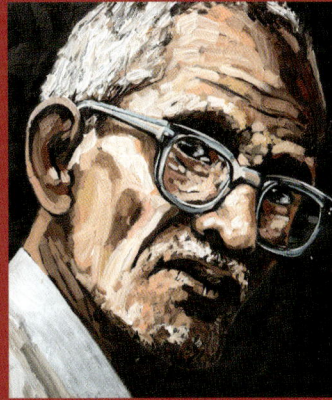

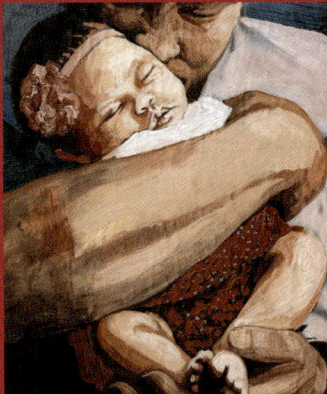

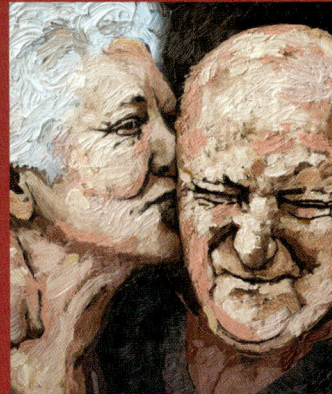

FROM THE VARIOUS interviews conducted to widen the range of our caregiving story connections, I have drawn from some more extensively than others in writing the chapters of this book. Several illustrations have given us only brief glimpses into the stories of the caregivers named, and some interviews have been held in reserve for this Treasury of Stories. I have chosen four stories to include here—two to expand and two to introduce—in hopes that you will find further affirmation, support, and insight to carry forward.

More About Donna's Story

Donna and Jim have two children: a son Nicholas, now 28 years old, and a daughter Natalie, a few years younger. Nicholas was born with multiple, severe disabilities. Cerebral palsy subjected him to exhausting pain; joint dislocations caused by bones growing faster than muscle created agonizing spasms. He has limited use of his limbs, great difficulty speaking, visual impairment, seizure disorder, nutritional challenges, and developmental delays.[1]

The level of care required to keep Nicholas alive, from the time of his birth to the present, is complex and extensive. The list of medical requirements for his care and the risks of failing to manage each task properly, cover nearly three pages of small print. As Nicholas grew up, Jim offered help when he could and was deeply engaged with his son's life, but with Jim's demanding full-time job that supported the family, the daily medical routines fell heavily to Donna in those years. Caring for Nicholas was profoundly exhausting, and little help was available. The Province of Ontario reimbursed certain expenses, but with 77 hospitalizations over Nicholas' life, and the need for 24/7 monitoring, the money did not go far. Donna used it mostly to hire high school students to help her son with homework so she could spend time with her daughter, or walk the dog, or make dinner. When Nicholas was healthy, he went to school, which gave Donna time to clean house or market for groceries. But when he was in long periods of pain or illness, her life was deeply isolated and she was seriously sleep deprived. Donna and Jim finally were able to get some night nursing help when Nicholas was 17, and at age 23 he moved into a care home where he still receives 24-hour one-to-one awake nursing care.

For all his physical disabilities and developmental delays, Nicholas is a very bright and determined young man. With the help of technology, he communicates using a set of head switches. In school he had the help of an educational assistant, a registered nurse, speech pathologists, occupational therapists, a physiotherapist, and a teacher of the visually impaired. Nicholas himself demonstrated extraordinary academic perseverance, keen memory, love of literature, and avid sports interests. Additionally, he has a fine sense of humor and a cheerful attitude in overcoming so much adversity. People love Nicholas, and he loves his life despite the enormous challenges he continues to face.

What enabled Donna to survive the 17 years in which she managed home care for Nicholas virtually by herself?

"Love!" is her immediate answer. "I adore my son, my daughter, my husband. It really is a combination of love and necessity. … Nicholas is nonspeaking, but he is so funny. He cracks jokes and I understand him just fine. There is a level of intimacy with people we look after. There are magical moments—sparks of living connection that we fan all the time just by giving care, by being together intimately. … It is a choice every day, a choice made because of love."

In her book, Donna describes the paradox that in order to be free, the mother of a child with severe disabilities has to relinquish most personal freedoms. She learned not to measure her family capacities "on the same scale as others—it is part of our job as people who love someone who is very dependent to redefine happiness and achievement."[2] Among the gifts Donna lifts up in her many years of caring for Nicholas, she notes, "I also understand deeply my own mortality and my interdependence. I have no illusion that I am an independent person. I learned how to accept that I needed help, and accept that other people want to help just like I want to give care. In this giving and receiving there is a balance of dignity and humility—and I think that is maturing."

Cyndy's Story

Employed by the mission outreach arm of a hospital system, Cyndy is an RN and faith community nurse who manages a health crisis intervention program in Colorado. She also has hospice training, which remains central to her perspectives and nursing practice. Cyndy and her husband, Tom, cared for their aged mothers for a period of about eight years, in a nearby retirement facility where both were located. Her mother passed away four-and-a-half years ago, and her mother-in-law about a year ago.

Asked about the most challenging aspects of her caregiving experience, Cyndy began with its sheer physicality. She is in her sixties now. While healthy, the challenge of getting wheelchairs and walkers in and out of cars—maneuvering them around wherever they needed to go—surprised her. She told a story of taking both mothers Christmas shopping one year—her mom in a wheelchair and Tom's on a walker with a seat. They had gotten through shopping and were waiting in the checkout line when Tom's mom began to feel faint. Cyndy got her seated on the walker and her nurse instincts immediately kicked in: she began to assess and monitor her mother-in-law's condition. "The poor people in line around us had no clue what to do with me," she laughed. "Then I was pushing the wheelchair and pulling the walker, along with all the things we had bought. Looking back, it was just comical—but also completely exhausting. Once I got us all back into the car, I thought, *Okay, I don't think I'll try that again!*"

As for emotional challenges, the greatest hurdle for Cyndy was feeling guilty for not being everything the two mothers wanted her to be. "My mother-in-law really wanted me to be her daughter; we absolutely loved and cared for each other, but you can't always be what someone needs you to be. With my mom it was similar: I could be her daughter and her favorite person in the world, but I couldn't be her *only* person in the world."

Guilt comes with feeling that no matter how much you do, it will never be enough. Cyndy and her husband both worked full-time and lived in a four-level house that would not have been a safe environment for their mothers to live in. Yet it can be hard to think you are doing enough, she admitted, "when you hear of others who quit their jobs, move, and do everything to accommodate their parents." Wisely, Cyndy came to accept that "it couldn't happen that way for me." She and Tom have four children and nine grandchildren. "It's a balancing act to take care of yourself, be a mom and a grandma, a daughter and a wife, along with full-time work. You just don't have unlimited time and energy and presence. I was taking away from one role to make another role happen."

Cyndy's initial act of self-care was accepting that she couldn't be everything to everyone. To bring balance to her various roles, she assessed her schedule—adding up her work hours along with eating and sleeping needs—then figured how much time she could realistically give their two mothers. She chose to focus on the quality rather than quantity of time spent with them: "When I was with them I gave them everything I could for that time, and helped them to stabilize emotionally." A significant learning was *to preserve a margin of space in her life for the unexpected*: the phone call at night reporting a fall, the ER visit, the days of hospitalization.

Spiritually, Cyndy understands that the guilt of feeling like we can never do or be enough does not come from God. It comes from our human nature. Learning to release self-judgment and let God be God has been one of her greatest lessons—one that she happily reports has transferred to other areas and relationships in her life.

The gifts Cyndy named in caregiving include developing patience, learning to breathe deeply through tough times, and experiencing the tenderness of intimate relationship with people in the end stages of life. She saw that God was in the moments of connection with their mothers—moments missed by family members who chose not to be involved: "When they share their history, their pain, a story that nobody else in the family has heard—but you hear it because you have built that trust and you are there, and they need to tell the story—their ability to go deeper into their lives with you is such a gift. You know God is present in these moments; it feels like a blessing specifically for you. And you are also participating in a healing presence for them as they tell a story they may never have told anyone."

Cyndy recognizes that in our last years, we all will have unresolved issues and memories we can't make sense of or haven't fully processed. Allowing ourselves to trust someone with that pain and confusion may help us realize that it is normal to feel the way we do. It can help us acknowledge our fears, and invite prayer or the assurance that God is with us no matter what we face.

Cyndy also learned, especially with her own mother, the importance of being truly heard. "I'm the oldest child, the one that is always in control. Just ask me and I will tell you how to do this—that's my personality! I had to reframe my way of listening to my mom, and learn to be fully with her. Instead of assuming I knew what she wanted, I had to truly listen to *her* tell me how she was feeling—her struggles, needs, and frustrations. I learned to listen without the mindset of fixing or having answers. I needed to communicate that I understood how tough this was for her, that I heard her pain even if I had no answers." It was a matter of simply respecting her mother's story for what it was and letting it stand.

Such a recognition lies at the root of Henri's image of the wounded healer. Cyndy identifies deeply with Henri's image: "We're always wounded, we're always healers; that's part of our humanity," she affirmed. "We have different stories but the same story. There are threads of humanity we can all connect to."

More About Vanessa's Story

Vanessa and Trey have two sons: Adam, now 18, is attending university, and Charlie, age 14, will soon enter eighth grade. Trey and Vanessa both work full-time jobs. Vanessa was a professor for many years and is currently engaged in university administration.

Charlie has a rare genetic disorder about which little is known. There is no prognosis and no care protocol for this condition. No support groups exist for parents of children afflicted by it. The symptoms mimic cerebral palsy in terms of physical coordination. Charlie has almost no control over his fine motor skills. He walks independently but awkwardly. He can use a keyboard slowly, but his fingers are so weak he cannot open a straw or package of food. Charlie's disabilities might have been limited to the physical but for a massive seizure he suffered at age three. Lasting over 45 minutes, it nearly cost his life. Long-duration seizures cause other body systems regulated by the brain, like heart and lungs, to shut down. Doctors surmised that Charlie's intellectual disabilities resulted from significant brain damage during that incident. The year following this trauma, the family moved to Nashville, where they could avail themselves of a children's hospital and epilepsy center.

Apart from early intervention specialists for his motor coordination issues, Vanessa and Trey had no home caregivers when Charlie was young. For a number of years now, Vanessa has had a friend babysit for Charlie every afternoon after school. She also comes overnight on those occasions when Vanessa and Trey travel for a few days. Charlie cannot be left entirely alone, and needs help cleaning himself up after trips to the bathroom. This less intensive care situation can be attributed in good measure to medical advances in treating Charlie's epilepsy. A neurologist in Nashville finally saw that the seizures were likely being triggered by migraine headaches, which in turn were caused by vascular tumors in Charlie's brain. In 2010, he was placed on an anti-migraine medication, after which his level of seizures decreased significantly.

For now, Charlie is stable, happy, loves his school, and is doing the best he can. He is verbal but shy, showing some characteristics associated with autism yet too empathetic to fit that diagnosis. He thrives with structured routines and loves flash card learning. Charlie has completed seventh grade, although he will never perform at grade level. His schooling consists of half mainstream classes and half special education classes. Charlie is with peers and absorbs as much as he is capable of learning. "I do not assume that he will qualify for a high school diploma," says Vanessa, "and that does not matter to me."

As children with disabilities get older, new challenges arise for their parents. A decision on the near horizon for Vanessa and Trey is where Charlie should go to high school. With increased concern about bullying, Trey feels strongly that a public high school would not be the right choice, whereas Vanessa does not want Charlie living away from them in a boarding school situation. Another option is a residential facility in Kentucky, where Charlie could experience community with others who have disabilities, reducing the level of stigma and perhaps opening up new possibilities for him. Vanessa's fondest dream would be for Charlie to live in a L'Arche community some day. (Of the two devotionals she uses daily, one is the Henri Nouwen Reader.) Charlie's parents cannot ask him to share his feelings about these options. While Charlie feels empathetically for others, he lacks the capacity to be cognitively self-reflective.

As Charlie moves into adolescence, another difficulty Vanessa describes is that her church community feels less and less like a place where she can find understanding or emotional support in relation to his needs. The differences between her two sons illustrate the challenge. The conversation she has with Adam's peer group of parents is all about which Ivy League schools the kids are getting into. But with Charlie's peer parents, she can't participate in such conversations, and it hurts. Charlie will not graduate from high school or go to college. He can't even go with the youth group on an overnight trip.

Another part of the story concerns Adam's relationship with Charlie and his parents. Vanessa knows that single siblings of a child with disabilities often put great pressure on themselves—perhaps to be everything their more limited siblings cannot be. Adam is a high achiever but also has a big heart, sticks up for the underdog, and is very willing to express compassion. Vanessa says Adam has always been thoughtful, yet she suspects his natural characteristics "have been encouraged by what he has seen us go through." Echoing other parents with a high-needs child among other children, Vanessa wishes she and Trey could have given more time and attention to Adam. "That is one of the hardest parts, especially now that he is in college," Vanessa muses. "But you cannot beat yourself up for that. I long for that lost time, but I also think you get what you get."

"I meditate," Vanessa says. "I am really comfortable with what I call 'sitting in the sad.' There are times when it is not about fixing it but just acknowledging the loneliness or sadness. It is really, really lonely. You are not alone, but it is lonely. I have to recognize that tension. It is not that I don't have friends; it is just that my friends do not have this path and have no way to understand it. I think people want to say or do the right thing, but they are really afraid of the realities of disability."

Tracy's Story

Tracy started her career as a probation officer. She had two young children when her mother was diagnosed with cancer at age 55. Her parents were divorced and Tracy lived in Minnesota near her father. But she quit her job and moved to California to be with her mother in the last six months of her mother's life under hospice care. Remarkably, Tracy's mother-in-law—who lived in Alaska—moved to California to support Tracy, caring for her two little ones while Tracy cared for her mom. Her mother-in-law had lost one son and didn't hesitate to "do what needed to be done" in this situation.

The experience of caring for her mother in those final months changed the direction of Tracy's life path, eventually taking her into hospice chaplaincy work. The circumstances around her mother's diagnosis were very distressing. Although her mom was in significant pain and attempted to get medical help more than 30 times over the course of a year, her primary care doctor made prejudicial assumptions and misdiagnosed her condition. In the presence of three of her mother's sisters, the doctor told her mother: "You are wasting your family's time and my time;

what you have is all in your head and you need to see a psychiatrist."
In fact, he wrote in her medical chart: "Black female—Demerol
seeker." He assumed Tracy's mother was a drug-seeker. His
labeling her was, in part, what kept ER doctors in her hometown
from ordering a simple ultrasound that would have found the
cancer. Tracy's mom went to stay with one of her sisters in Reno,
Nevada. There she managed to see another doctor who did order
an ultrasound and found tumors everywhere. The cancer was
already at Stage 4.

Tracy's mom was transported back to California and placed
under hospice care. At that point, Tracy said, "All that mattered
was taking care of her and making her comfortable. There was
just no room for working through my feelings about the
misdiagnosis and how long Mom had suffered from such
unnecessary pain."

Despite the circumstances, profound gifts emerged for Tracy
from that six-month period of caring for her mom. "When you
are confronted with the reality of a known time limit to life, the
richness of that life really comes forward. It's as if being in that
space magnified the color and richness of the conversation.
There's a lot of reminiscing, contemplating what matters, being
aware of what needs to be expressed. I recall the joy on Mom's
face talking about her sweet potato pie recipe, the emotion in
her hands showing how she used the nutmeg. Those memories
had more vibrancy, so many layers. That sense of connection—
who we are and what we mean to each other—just can't be
manufactured." Tracy saw that "caregiving allowed for a place
of healing"—not physically, but her mom had confidence in
Tracy's care for her and felt very safe, which added a deeper level
of comfort.

After her mother's death, Tracy returned home and focused
on her own growing family. She and her husband adopted three

children at one time, then had another biological child—six children in all. But her experience with her mom's care had deeply impacted her. She volunteered with a hospital chaplain and knew deep down that God was calling her to this kind of work. Over the course of her training, she worked alternately between hospital and hospice chaplaincy settings.

When an opportunity came for full-time hospice work, Tracy asked her youngest son—12 at the time—what he thought. His reply: "Well, I think you're more of a hospice dying-chaplain than a hospital dying-chaplain. When you talk about the way people die at the hospital, it's always a really bad experience, but when you talk about people dying in hospice, you almost smile!" Tracy says all her kids have a different understanding of life because of her chaplaincy work.

The gifts she felt while caring for her mom continue to feed Tracy's work as a chaplain. She steps back into the richness of the experience, the sense of gift and healing, as she accompanies others through the tender time of knowing a distinct limit to a loved one's life. Being with others this way allows the continued healing of her own memories, especially the difficult ones related to her mother's suffering.

Fifteen years after her mother's death, Tracy had the opportunity to put into practice her hospice learning and experience with her father. He was 85 years old when the diagnosis came, and he opted not to undergo treatment his doctor said was worse than the disease. Tracy was the adult child her father trusted most, as she had lived near him for 15 years in Minnesota after her parents' divorce. Tracy cared for him from a distance, flying from Colorado to Minnesota every two weeks until he needed more intensive care: "The diagnosis set him in a place where he really wanted to express his heart, and I was blessed to be present for him to do that."

In caring for her mom, Tracy had tried to "be strong" for her sake and her grandmother's sake. Looking back, she realized it was not true strength, as it robbed her of self-care. Tracy engaged in better self-care while supporting her dad. She allowed herself to grieve his loss before his death: "I let myself be present with whatever I was feeling. So I talked more and reached out more for support."

As a hospice chaplain, she gives family caregivers permission to step back and see their exhaustion, even their irritability with a loved one, as normal. "Caregiving at the end of life is such an emotional journey. People often don't realize how heavy the work is, not just physically, but emotionally and spiritually. The balance comes in paying attention to all those parts; talking and valuing where you are emotionally, and connecting with your resources like a chaplain, friend, or pastor." During her mother's illness, Tracy's home church was very supportive, picking up her traveling husband from the airport, bringing meals, and simply being present when she needed to express anger at God over her mother's situation. Her mother-in-law also encouraged her not to hide her feelings from God: "He knows already, so don't put that wall between you!" was her message. Tracy brings these insights into her hospice ministry now. "We are called to bear one another's burdens, and so fulfill the law of Christ. That law is loving one another. It is a *gift* you offer someone else to say, 'I need you to bear this burden with me.'"

Further Resources

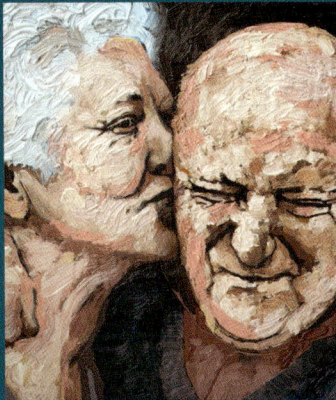

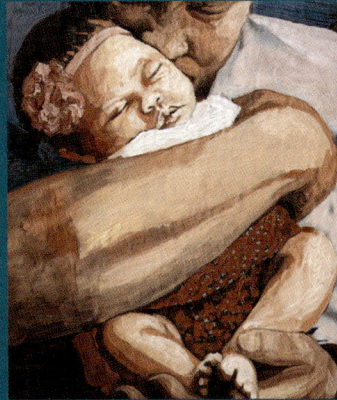

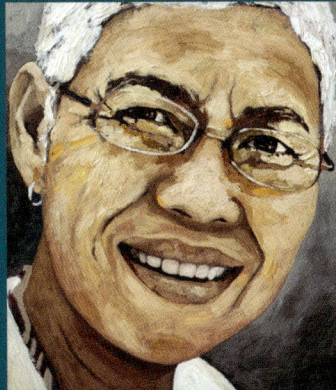

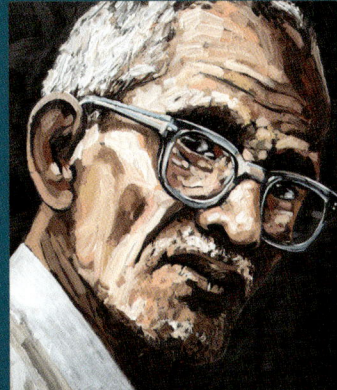

Morning and Evening Prayer for Retreat

MORNING PRAYER (10 MINUTES)

SONG — Select from your available hymnals or songbooks; 1–2 verses

PSALM — Select one: Psalm 13, 42, or 77:1–15. These psalms give voice to the suffering side of life. Read without haste; or create a psalm handout and read in unison.

SILENCE — Invite a brief time of quiet for participants to reflect on a phrase or image from the psalm that spoke to them.

PRAYER — Aim to help caregivers release their anxieties and be present to the gifts of this day. The prayer should be only a few minutes.

BLESSING — A traditional benediction or one of your own.

EVENING PRAYER (10 MINUTES)

SONG — If you have access to Taizé chants or Iona Community songs, they are excellent for retreat settings; or choose one or two verses of an evening hymn.

PSALM — Recommended: Psalm 23, 63:1–8, or 84. These psalms voice the experience of solace, comfort, blessing and joy.

PRAYER — Gather thanks and praise for the insights and blessings of the day. Pray yourself, or invite one-sentence prayers from participants.

BLESSING — Traditional or spontaneous.

Please Listen to Me

When I ask you to listen to me
and you start giving me advice
you have not done what I asked.

When I ask you to listen to me
and you begin to tell me why I shouldn't feel that way
you are telling me to deny my feelings.

When I ask you to listen to me
and you feel you have to do something to solve my problems,
you have failed me (strange as that may seem).

Listen.

All I ask is that you listen.

Not talk or do
—just hear me.
The giving of advice
can never take the place
of the giving of yourself.

I'm not helpless, or hopeless!

When you do something for me
that I need to do for myself
you contribute to my fear
… and weakness.

But when you accept
the simple fact that I do feel what I feel
(no matter how irrational that may seem to you),
then I quit trying to convince you
and can get on with
trying to understand
what's behind my feelings.

And when that's clear,
the answers are obvious.
And you know what?
Your listening made that possible.

—Anonymous

This content was published in Courage for Caregivers: Sustenance for the Journey in Company with Henri J. M. Nouwen *by Marjorie J. Thompson (Church Health and Henri Nouwen Society, 2017). Permission to reproduce for non-commercial ministry use.*

Writing Letters

Henri Nouwen was a prolific letter writer. He kept up an amazing volume of correspondence with hundreds of individuals over his lifetime. Some were ordinary letters to family or friends, but many were letters of spiritual guidance and support written to people struggling with painful questions and circumstances. An entire volume of Henri's letters have now been published in a book entitled, *Love, Henri.** The title reflects how he signed his name.

It is rare that people today take time to write letters by hand. Yet writing a letter can be a fine way to express your own questions, feelings, story fragments, and insights. People who keep a regular journal sometimes think of it as an extended letter to themselves, or to someone who might eventually read their words, or even to God. Letters to family and close friends are not usually formal compositions, but rather spontaneous expressions of what we are experiencing and thinking. Like personal journals, they don't need to be grammatically correct or even written in complete sentences!

Writing a letter can be a very useful tool to reflect, process life, or express difficult feelings. It can be equally helpful to caregivers and care receivers capable of writing. To whom do you wish to write? Some appropriate options, given the topic of this book, would include: God; yourself; your care receiver (or caregiver); a family member; a loved one who has died; Henri Nouwen.

Guidelines: be honest; speak your heart; say what you want and need to say. Such letters need not be sent, but if you plan to send one take kindness into account.

---

*Love, Henri, *copyright by The Henri Nouwen Legacy Trust, was published by Convergent Books, an imprint of Crown Publishing Group, in 2016.*

This content was published in Courage for Caregivers: Sustenance for the Journey in Company with Henri J. M. Nouwen *by Marjorie J. Thompson (Church Health and Henri Nouwen Society, 2017). Permission to reproduce for non-commercial ministry use.*

A Meditation for Compassionate Self-observation

Each of us has, deep inside, the capacity to see with eyes of compassion. Christ, who indwells our heart, sees with love. With a little intention and practice we can access our heart-center in daily life. Here is one way to practice compassion for ourselves. Get in touch with something about yourself you really dislike and wish you could be rid of—perhaps a character weakness or bad habit. Become aware of your usual feelings in relation to this. Notice the feelings without sinking too deeply into them.

Now take a step back from your judging ego to a deeper center, a place of interior freedom from which you can observe your reactions and feelings. This is your inner sanctuary of love, where the compassionate Spirit burns like a little pilot light.

Breathe and relax into this heart-center. Just as oxygen feeds a flame, let your breath feed the Spirit-flame within, till it is full and bright. Feel compassion fill your heart.

From this compassionate center, look at the part of yourself you so dislike. What do you observe?

Let the compassionate One in your heart give comfort to the wounded child in you—with words, or song, or a gesture of embrace. Notice how your inner child responds.

Accept a higher love for yourself—even in weakness, brokenness, and incompletion.

You are a work in progress. Christ bears with you patiently.

Take a moment now to name and absorb the gift of this meditation.

This content was published in Courage for Caregivers: Sustenance for the Journey in Company with Henri J. M. Nouwen *by Marjorie J. Thompson (Church Health and Henri Nouwen Society, 2017). Permission to reproduce for non-commercial ministry use.*

Observing Another with Compassion

The "Indwelling Spirit" or "true self" in our deepest heart sees with the eyes of compassion. With a little intention and practice we can access this center in daily life.

Suppose someone says or does something that makes you feel irritated, embarrassed, anxious, or offended. Instead of letting your typical reactions take you over, try this:

Take a deep breath, step back inwardly, and name what you are feeling. Rather than closing off the person who has offended, keep your heart open.

Take a second breath and go deeper inside. Find the Heart of your heart, a place of compassion within you that burns like a gentle flame. Feel the warmth of care and concern in this deep center.

By imagination, "feed the flame" with your breathing—just as airflow increases the intensity of a fire. See the light, feel the warmth swelling as you allow your loving intention to grow.

From the lighted eyes of compassion, look now on this person. What do you see? Can you discern some need, suffering, ignorance, or immaturity behind the offending words or behavior?

Let the compassion of Christ guide you. Allow your response to this person to arise from this deep center—whether in silent thought, imagined act, or spoken words.

Take a few moments after to write down what you noticed as a compassionate observer, and what insight you receive from this process.

Meditations developed by Marjorie Thompson with reference to ideas and processes borrowed from Jane Vennard. Permission to reproduce with the following attribution.

*"The Compassionate Observer" is a phrase coined by Jane Vennard. See A Praying Congregation: The Art of Teaching Spiritual Practice *(Alban Institute, 2005, 99-100). These meditations differ significantly from Vennard's original exercises. The borrowed phrase and a few of her images are used with Vennard's permission.*

Dying Well

Death is a subject we often resist talking about openly. We live in a culture that is deeply uncomfortable with death, despite the fact that daily news is full of it and we all know perfectly well that every one of us will die at some point. We are afraid of death just as we are afraid of pain and suffering. Because we cannot control or predict our dying, we feel helpless before it. It often seems easier to avoid or ignore the fact that death lurks in the background of life.

The losses of death touch everyone sooner or later. Yet caring for those who are weak, disabled, seriously ill, or elderly puts us in a position of facing the probabilities of death sooner rather than later. How do we become more comfortable thinking and talking together about our dying? What promises of faith support and guide us as we do this?

Henri Nouwen grappled with death and dying as a spiritual challenge and wrote a good deal on the subject, particularly after his mother's death; after his own brush with death from a roadside accident; and after the deaths of several "core members" of the L'Arche Daybreak community—core members being those with developmental disabilities, like Adam, whom he cared for daily. Henri studied psychology early in his ministry, and discovered the phrase "befriending death" in the work of Carl Jung. He came to believe that it is important for us to "befriend our death" and thus allow it to become fruitful in the lives of others. Following are several illuminating concepts from Henri's writings on this subject.

WISDOM FROM HENRI ON BEFRIENDING DEATH AND DYING AS GIFT

- Since we all will die, can our death become something more than an unavoidable fate? Might death be seen an act of fulfillment?
- Just as we prepare for the birth of a child, can we prepare attentively for our death? Could we anticipate death as a friend waiting to welcome us home?
- We can befriend death. But first we must claim that we are children of God.
- Death is not the end of our fruitfulness. Life bears fruit long after it has come to an end. (Read more on these ideas in *Our Greatest Gift: A Meditation on Dying and Caring.*)

- Believing that you were beloved before you were born makes it possible to realize life is a mission. In the years of your life, can you help others know they are beloved as well? (This concept is from the "*Befriending Death*" address.)
- It is important to be prepared for death, and not wait until we are close to death to begin reflecting on it. (Henri wrote about this in *A Letter of Consolation*.)
- When death comes near, what we say or write to people who are close to us can make our deaths a gift for others. How do we express gratitude, forgiveness, grace? (Henri reflects on making our deaths a gift in *Bread for the Journey*, meditation for May 16.)

WISDOM FROM MICHELLE O'ROURKE, PALLIATIVE CARE NURSE

Michelle O'Rourke, a palliative care nurse and coordinator at a residential hospice, has this to say about those whose lives touch death and dying:

"It simply comes down, sooner or later, to how comfortable you are with yourself, with others, and with the whole idea of dying and grief, because working with those affected by death and bereavement often involves more 'being' than doing."

If we want to be helpful as caregivers to those who are near to death, there are several things to be aware of. For a person to die well takes some time and preparation. Here are elements that need attention, according to O'Rourke:

- Coming to terms with the diagnosis—patient and family
- "Living" until you die
- Relationship completion
- Unfinished business
- Legacy work
- Hope and healing

Coming to terms with the diagnosis, if you have time to do so, involves moving through many experiences of grief and loss.

Living until you die is what life is always about! "Palliative care is about helping people to live the final and perhaps most important part of their life's journey well."

Dr. Ira Byock says the five most important things to say for Relationship Completion are:

- "I forgive you." (Forgiveness)
- "Forgive me." (Reconciliation)
- "Thank you." (Gratitude)
- "I love you." (Love)
- "Goodbye." (Mystery)

Unfinished business can be unresolved relational issues, important conversations still needed to bring peace to the dying and their loved ones, or practical matters.

Legacy work may involve financial disbursements, decisions about how to preserve life achievements, or express more of a personal legacy of memories and values to one's family or community.

Hope and healing become emotional and spiritual matters for one who is dying. Relational healing is key, both with others and with God. Spiritual healing may revolve around anger, doubt, loneliness, feeling abandoned by God, fear of judgment, or anxiety around one's life purpose or meaning.

Substantial elements of this section are drawn from Embracing the End of Life: Help for Those Who Accompany the Dying *by Michelle O'Rourke and Eugene DuFour Novalis Publishing Inc., 2012).*

This content was published in Courage for Caregivers: Sustenance for the Journey in Company with Henri J. M. Nouwen *by Marjorie J. Thompson (Church Health and Henri Nouwen Society, 2017). Permission to reproduce for non-commercial ministry use.*

Congregational Support
for Caregivers

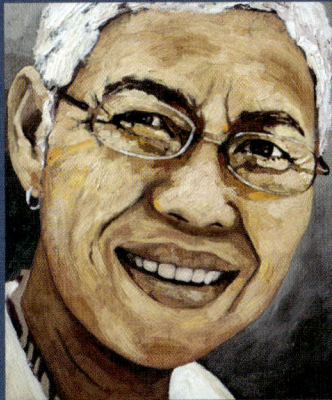

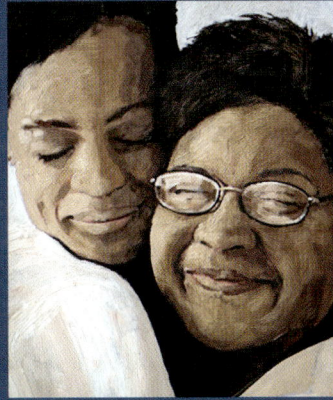

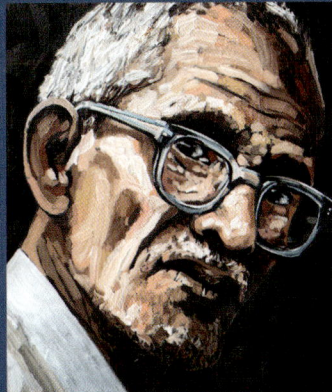

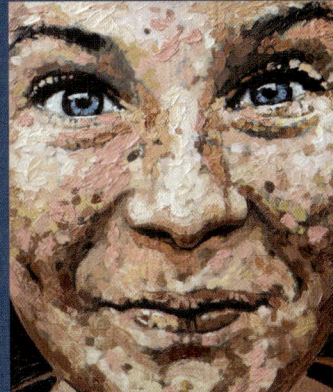

Enabling Caregivers to Attend Retreats

While some caregiver schedules allow for greater participation in church, school, or community events, many find the relentlessness of their responsibilities so consuming that even one retreat day apart is difficult to arrange. Congregational leaders who hope to serve their caregivers well will need to exercise determination and creativity to maximize participation, especially for those who need it most.

A few possibilities to consider:

- Arrange for supervised "adult care" at the church during the planned retreat, just as childcare is often provided to enable busy parents to attend events. Since a church cannot offer trained nursing care, the level of help required by care receivers will naturally limit who could benefit from this offering. However, such adult care might be appropriate for seniors with mobility issues or less severe memory limitations, as well as people of various ages with milder intellectual disabilities.
- An adequate number of supervising adults to help with various needs must be considered. These people would need to be carefully selected, with a reasonable level of experience in the issues faced by the care receivers.
- Church facilities, especially handicapped-accessible bathrooms, would need to be taken into account.
- Develop a church fund earmarked for respite care, particularly for those caregivers whose tasks are more complex and whose care receivers need levels of expertise that prevent them from easily leaving home. The funds could be offered for additional hours of in-home care support, allowing caregivers time away for a day apart.

Offering Respite Care Volunteers

As a society we are only beginning to wake up and count the

real cost of caregiving. We have begun to recognize the value of time, energy, and love expended for the sake of those who need care—and the physical, emotional, and spiritual cost to caregivers over long years in this role. The challenge of supporting caregivers at home is surfacing as a major issue, nationally and around the world. As people live longer and populations age, the care needs of those with Alzheimer's, other forms of dementia, chronic illness, or other disabilities will only increase over time. We are becoming more aware of the issues faced by people of many ages with serious brain injuries from combat, professional sports, or accidents. The situations and needs are varied and complex. Many home caregivers have been virtually invisible to society at large.

Family caregivers are often under great financial stress. What might it look like for faith communities to begin training a cadre of respite care volunteers? Again, this ministry would not take on highly skilled care needs, but rather the kind of needs many home care agencies offer, such as meal preparation, light housekeeping, help with toileting, and simple companionship.

Such volunteers could enable family caregivers to get out for much needed recreation and self-care—a few hours of rest and personal enjoyment without the added expense of professional home caregivers.

Caregiver Support Groups

One largely unmet need is the opportunity for caregivers to meet with a support group. Caregivers who feel deeply isolated need to know they are not alone. They need a safe place to share feelings, hopes, and questions, trusting they will be heard and not judged. Again, some caregivers' responsibilities are not overly burdensome and allow a measure of freedom to attend gatherings. As we find creative ways to support those with greater burdens, we can more effectively offer them such opportunities as well.

APPENDIX E

Pastoral care ministers, chaplains, nurses, social workers, or therapists could all be helpful leaders of support groups. Laypersons with past experience in caregiving might also lead effectively. Such groups could benefit from periodically bringing in people with particular expertise in areas like grief work, self-care, creative expression, or spiritual practice.

Online Resources

Many caregivers who cannot easily get out of their homes at least have access to the Internet, and thus to various forms of online support. Faith communities can add sections to their websites on caregiving, with bibliographies, blogposts, video libraries— even online support groups and online workshops. Facebook and other social media also provide group platforms for interactive support.

We hope many of the resources listed in this book will be helpful in the development of such web-based congregational support to caregivers.

Print and Video Resources

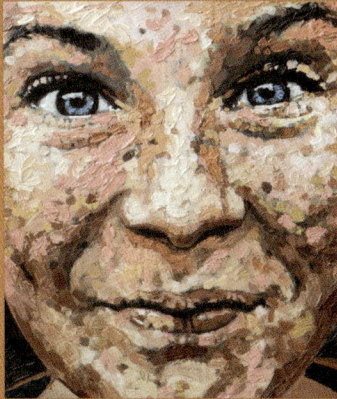

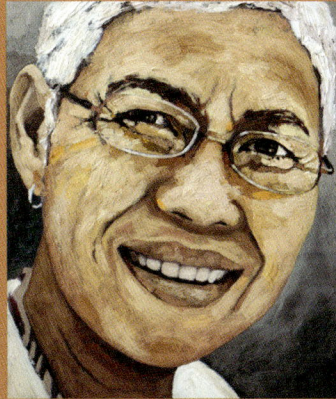

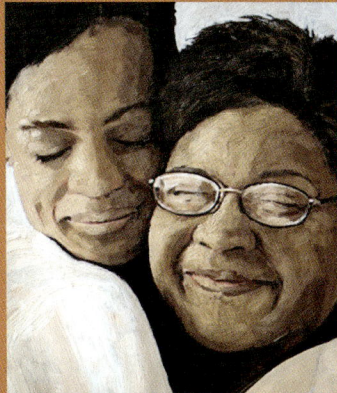

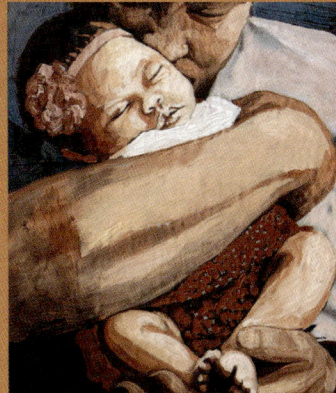

Henri Nouwen Publications Cited in Courage for Caregivers:

"Care and the Elderly," Pamphlet adapted from speech delivered June 6, 1975

Our Greatest Gift: A Meditation on Dying and Caring (Harper San Francisco, 1994)

A *Spirituality of Caregiving*, Ed. John S. Mogabgab (Upper Room Books, 2011)

Life of the Beloved: Spiritual Living in a Secular World (Crossroad, 1992)

The Road to Peace (Orbis, 1998)

Can You Drink the Cup? (Ave Maria Press, 1996)

Adam: God's Beloved (Orbis, 1997)

The Wounded Healer (Image Books, 1979)

With Burning Hearts, (Orbis, 1994)

Bread for the Journey (Harper San Francisco, 1997)

Letters to Marc About Jesus (Darton, Longman and Todd, 1988)

Return of the Prodigal Son (Doubleday, 1992)

Finding My Way Home (Crossroad, 2004)

Here and Now (Crossroad, 1999)

The Way of the Heart (Seabury Press, 1981)

Other Relevant Nouwen Books:

Beyond the Mirror: Reflections on Death and Life (Crossroad, 1990)

In Memoriam (Ave Maria Press, 1980)

Turn My Mourning into Dancing: Finding Hope in Hard Times (W Publishing Group, Thomas Nelson, 2001)

The Inner voice of Love: A Journey Through Anguish to Freedom (Image Books, Doubleday, 1998)

McNeil, Morrison and Nouwen, *Compassion: A Reflection on the Christian Life* (Doubleday & Co, 1992)

Love, Henri (Convergent Books, an imprint of Crown Publishing Group, 2016)

Other Book Resources

Brené Brown, *The Gifts of Imperfection* (Hazelden Publishing, 2010)

Ira Byock, *Dying Well: Peace and Possibilities at the End of Life* (Penguin, 1998)

Ira Byock, *The Four Things That Matter Most* (10th Anniversary Edition (Atria Books, 2014)

Ron DelBene, *Into the Light: A Way to Pray with the Sick and Dying* (Wipf and Stock, 2009)

Christopher deVinck, *The Power of the Powerless: A Brother's Lessons* (Doubleday, 1990)

Michelle O'Rourke, *Befriending Death: Henri Nouwen and a Spirituality of Dying* (Orbis Books, 2009)

Michelle O'Rourke and Eugene Dufour, *Embracing the End of Life: Help for Those Who Accompany the Dying* (Novalis Publishing Inc., 2012)

Donna Thomson, *The Four Walls of My Freedom: Lessons I've Learned from a Life of Caregiving* (House of Anansi Press, Toronto, Ontario, 2010)

Saki Santorelli, *Heal Thy Self: Lessons on Mindfulness in Medicine* (Bell Tower, a division of Crown Publishing 1999)

Videos

"Behind the Glass Door"—One family's struggle with the mysterious and debilitating disorder of autism. This is part of Hannah's story, produced in 2001 by Windborne Productions (Markham, Ontario) and available for purchase at www.windborneproductions.com.

"Impoverished Places"—DVD of Judy's dance—a woman suffering from Parkinson's, enabled to express her inner life with the help of a professional dancer. Produced by Windborne Productions, this short video is available for purchase at www.windborneproductions.com.

Endnotes

Beginnings

1. Henri J. M. Nouwen, *Here and Now: Living in the Spirit* (Crossroad, 1994), 144.
2. Henri J. M. Nouwen, "Care and the Elderly," Pamphlet adapted from a speech delivered June 6, 1975 (The Henri Nouwen Legacy Trust, 2008), 5.
3. Henri J. M. Nouwen, *Our Greatest Gift: A Meditation on Dying and Caring* (Harper San Francisco, 1994), 51-52.

Chapter 1
The Mutuality of Caregiving:
Shared Suffering and Compassion

1. "Care and the Elderly," 3.
2. "Care and the Elderly," 4.
3. "Care and the Elderly," 4.
4. "Care and the Elderly," 7.
5. Henri J. M. Nouwen, *A Spirituality of Caregiving*, Ed. John S. Mogabgab (Upper Room Books, 2011), p. 16.
6. "Care and the Elderly," 6.
7. Henri J. M. Nouwen, Walk With Jesus: Stations of the Cross (Orbis Books, 1990). Cited in *A Spirituality of Caregiving*, 18.
8. *A Spirituality of Caregiving*, 19.
9. Henri J. M. Nouwen, *Can You Drink the Cup?* (Ave Maria Press, 1996), 35-36.
10. Henri J. M. Nouwen, *Can You Drink the Cup?* (Ave Maria Press, 1996), 37.
11. *A Spirituality of Caregiving*, 16-17.
12. *A Spirituality of Caregiving*, 24-25.
13. See Henri J. M. Nouwen, *Adam: God's Beloved* (Orbis, 1997), 78-79.
14. Christopher deVinck, *The Power of the Powerless: A Brother's Lessons* (Doubleday, 1990).
15. *The Wounded Healer* (Image Books, 1979) was one of Henri's most celebrated early works and remains a classic.
16. *A Spirituality of Caregiving*, 52.
17. *A Spirituality of Caregiving*, 31.

Chapter 2

The Challenges of Caregiving

1. *A Spirituality of Caregiving*, 17.
2. *A Spirituality of Caregiving*, 33.
3. A description of the five elements of Relationship Completion and other aspects of dying well can be found in Appendix D. These concepts are explored in Dr. Ira Byock's book, *Dying Well: The Prospect of Growth at the End of Life* (Penguin, 1998).
4. *A Spirituality of Caregiving*, 26.
5. *A Spirituality of Caregiving*, 38-39.

Chapter 3

The Gifts of Caregiving: Seeing and Celebrating

1. Sue Mosteller, C. S. J., Henri's literary executrix.
2. "From sermon, "Being the Beloved," delivered 8/22/92 on the Hour of Power" program.
3. From an audio-taped address titled "Caring," Hilton Head Island Spiritual Formation Emphasis Week, Evening Community Session at St. Francis, 10/6/93.
4. *Our Greatest Gift*, xiii.
5. *A Spirituality of Caregiving*, 39.
6. From an unpublished journal entry dated 3/2/86 (cited in *Seeds of Hope*, Ed. Robert Durback, Bantam Books, 1989), 147.

7. Lawrence Calhoun and Richard Tedeschi of the University of North Carolina at Charlotte, cited in "Grief and Gratitude" by Lynne Steuerle Schofield, Swarthmore College Bulletin, Winter 2016, p. 4.
8. Henri J. M. Nouwen, *The Return of the Prodigal Son* (Doubleday, 1992), 117.
9. From Henri J. M. Nouwen, "The Path of Living and Dying," in *Finding My Way Home*, (Crossroad Publishing Company, 2004), 79.
10. Reid Ward, in a communication to friends from early 2016. Used with permission.
11. Rev. Gordon Peerman, homily preached January 14, 2017. Used by permission.
12. *The Return of the Prodigal Son*, 75 and 119.

Chapter 4

The Sustenance of Caregiving: Self-care and Spiritual Practice

1. Parker J. Palmer, *Let Your Life Speak: Listening for the Voice of Vocation* (Jossey-Bass, 2000), 30.
2. Michelle O'Rourke and Eugene Dufour, *Embracing the End of Life: Help for Those Who Accompany the Dying* (Novalis Publishing Inc., 2012), 143. Emphasis added.
3. The two questions and first list are adapted from PowerPoint slides O'Rourke

permission.

4. The second list and point about presence are drawn from an interview with Henri Nouwen, University of Notre Dame Alumni, Continuing Education, April 3, 1996.

5. See O'Rourke and Dufour, *Embracing the End of Life*, 141-142.

6. Brené Brown, *The Gifts of Imperfection* (Hazelden Publishing, 2010), p. 20, abridged.

7. From "Befriending Death," an address to the National Catholic AIDS Network, Chicago, July 1995.

8. Ron Rolheiser, OMI, "Helping Simon of Cyrene Carry Jesus' Cross," abridged from meditation dated 3/10/17 on website: http://ronrolheiser.com/helping-simon-of-cyrene-carry-jesus-cross-4-of-6/#.WOF1IhArLrc. Used by permission.

9. Attributed to the Greek-speaking Stoic philosopher Epictetus, 55-135 AD.

10. See Appendix D for resources on listening that could be used as handouts.

11. For more on Breath Prayer, see Ron DelBene, *Into the Light: A Way to Pray with the Sick and Dying* (Wipf and Stock, 2009).

12. Henri J. M. Nouwen, *The Way of the Heart* (Seabury Press, 1981), 82.

13. Abridged from a lecture at Scarritt-Bennett Center in Nashville, TN, 2/8/91.

Appendix C: A Treasury of Stories

1. Description adapted from Donna Thomson's book, *The Four Walls of My Freedom* (The House of Anansi Press, 2014), 137.

2. Donna Thomson, 87.

FEATURED INSPIRATIONAL QUOTES
Beginnings

Page 21: Saki Santorelli, *Heal Thy Self: Lessons on Mindfulness in Medicine* (Bell Tower, 1999), 20

Chapter 1

Page 23: Henri Nouwen, *Life of the Beloved: Spiritual Living in a Secular World* (Crossroad Publishing Company, 1992; 10th Anniversary ed., 2002), 97.

Page 24: Henri J. M. Nouwen, "Christ of Americas" (America Magazine, April 21, 1984) in The Road to Peace (Orbis, 1998), 111.

Page 27: Henri J. M. Nouwen, *Can You Drink the Cup?* (Ave Maria Press, 1996), 38.

Chapter 2

Page 37: Madeleine L'Engle, *A Rock that Is Higher* (A Shaw Book: Published by WaterBrook Press, Colorado Springs, CO, 2002), 220.

Page 40: Henri J. M. Nouwen, *With Burning Hearts* (Orbis, 1994), 32.

Page 43: Henri J. M. Nouwen, *Bread for the Journey*, Meditation for Jan 5. (HarperSanFrancisco, 1997).

Page 46: Henri J. M. Nouwen, *Our Greatest Gift: A Meditation on Dying and Caring* (HarperSan Francisco, 1994), 14.

Chapter 3

Page 52: Henri J. M. Nouwen, *Letters to Marc About Jesus* (Darton, Longman and Todd, 1988), 60.

Page 57: From "Befriending Death" address to the National Catholic AIDS Network, Chicago, July 1995.

Chapter 4

Page 74: Henri J. M. Nouwen, *Our Greatest Gift: A Meditation on Dying and Caring* (HarperSan Francisco, 1994), 63.

Page 76: Henri J. M. Nouwen, *Here and Now: Living in the Spirit* (Crossroad Publishing Company, 1999), 109-110 abridged.

Page 82: Rachel Naomi Remen, *Kitchen Table Wisdom: Stories That Heal* (The Penguin Group, New York, NY, 1996, 2006), 143-144.

Page 88: Madeleine L'Engle, *Walking on Water: Reflections on Faith and Art* (Convergent Books, an imprint of Crown Publishing Group, a division of Penguin Random House LLC, New York, 2016), 182.

Page 89: Deborah Hunsinger, "Keeping an Open Heart in Troubled Times," in *A Spiritual Life: Perspectives from Poets, Prophets, and Preachers*, Ed. Allan Hugh Cole, Jr. (Westminster John Knox Press, 2011), 127.

Permissions

Grateful acknowledgement is made for permission to reprint the following excerpts from previously published works by Henri J. M. Nouwen.

Excerpts from *A Spirituality of Caregiving*, by Henri J. M. Nouwen, copyright © 2011 by the Henri Nouwen Legacy Trust. Used by permission of the Henri Nouwen Legacy Trust. Published by Upper Room Books.

Excerpts from *Seeds of Hope: A Henri Nouwen Reader*, copyright © 1997 by Robert Durback, is reprinted by permission of the Henri Nouwen Legacy Trust. Originally published in 1989 by Penguin Random House.

Excerpt from *Care and the Elderly*, by Henri J. M. Nouwen, copyright © 2008 by the Henri Nouwen Legacy Trust, is reprinted by permission of the Henri Nouwen Legacy Trust.

Excerpts from *Bread for the Journey: A Daybook of Wisdom and Faith*, by Henri J. M. Nouwen, copyright © 1997 by the Henri Nouwen Legacy Trust. Reprinted courtesy of HarperCollins Publishers.

Excerpts from *Letters to Marc About Jesus* by Henri J. M. Nouwen, copyright ©1987, 1988 by Henri J. M. Nouwen. English translation copyright © 1988 by Harper and Row Publishers Inc. and Darton, Longman & Todd, Ltd. Reprinted courtesy of HarperCollins Publishers.

Excerpts from *Our Greatest Gift: A Meditation on Dying and Caring*, by Henri J. M. Nouwen, copyright © 1994 by Henri J. M. Nouwen. Reprinted courtesy of HarperCollins Publishers.

Excerpt from *The Gifts of Imperfection: Let Go of Who You Think You're Supposed to Be and Embrace Who You Are*, by Brené Brown, published in 2010, is courtesy of Hazelden Publishers.

Excerpt from *Heal Thy Self: Lessons on Mindfulness in Medicine*, by Saki Santorelli, published in 2000, is courtesy of Penguin Random House LLC. All rights reserved.

Excerpt from *Kitchen Table Wisdom*, by Rachel Naomi Remen, published in 1996, is courtesy of Penguin Random House LLC. All rights reserved.

Excerpt from *Walking on Water: Reflections on Faith and Art*, by Madeleine L'Engle, published in 2001, is courtesy of Penguin Random House LLC. All rights reserved.

Excerpt from *The Rock that is Higher*, by Madeleine L'Engle, published in 2002, is courtesy of Penguin Random House LLC. All rights reserved.

Excerpt from *Let Your Life Speak: Listening to the Voice of Vocation*, by Parker J. Palmer, published in 1999, is courtesy of Jossey-Boss Education Publishers, a Wiley imprint. Copyright 2000 by John Wiley and Sons, Inc. All rights reserved.

Excerpt from *Embracing the End of Life: Help for Those Who Accompany the Dying* by Michelle O'Rourke and Eugene Dufour, published in 2013, is courtesy of Novalis Publishing.

Excerpt from *Keeping an Open Heart in Troubled Times*, by Deborah Hunsinger, was published in A Spiritual Life: Perspectives from Poets, Prophets and Preachers, ed. Allan Hugh Cole Jr., 2011, and is courtesy of Westminster John Knox Press.

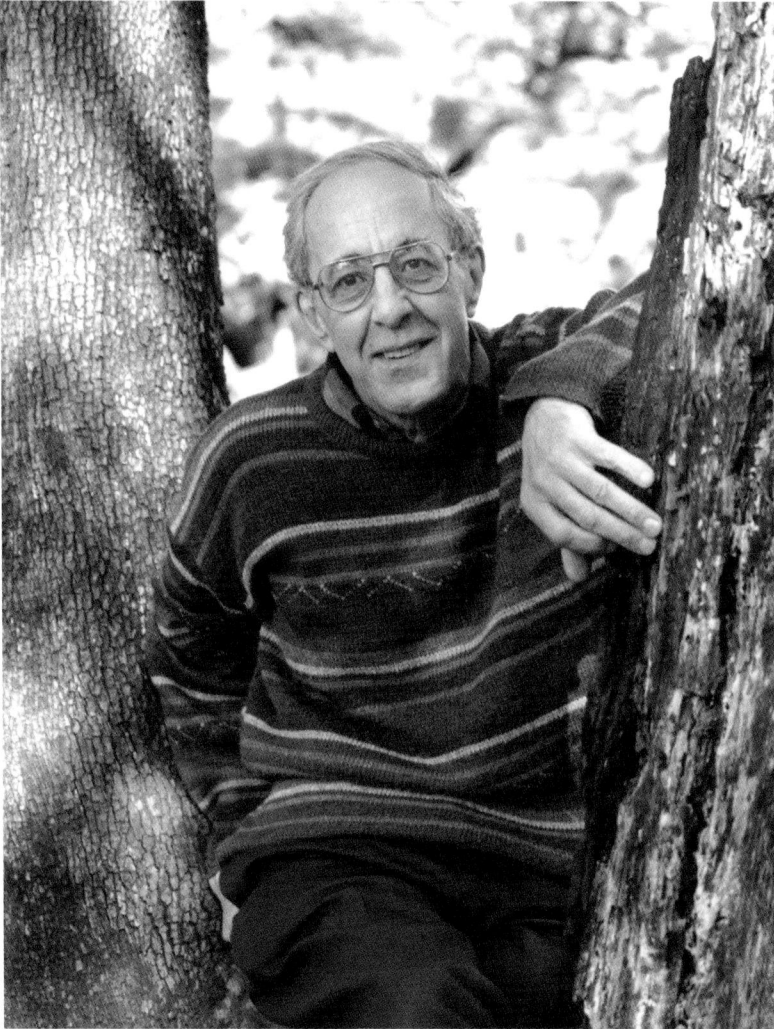

HENRI J. M. NOUWEN

1932–1996

Marjorie Thompsons's authoring of Courage for Caregivers is a unique and rich contribution to the "vocation," of caregiving, which Marjorie knows both as freely chosen and as accepted in loving duty. Schooled by Henri Nouwen at Yale, and by her mother and her mother-in-law through years of caregiving, Marjorie allowed her teachers to gift her with inner transformation on the journey toward deep integrity and compassion. This transformation is evident in the wide-ranging vision of caregiving offered here. Added to her personal growth and insights are the gifts and challenges of others in caregiving situations, along the spiritual perceptions of a lifelong pastor and friend to the suffering, Henri Nouwen. Marjorie Thompson has profound gifts for feeling, discerning, and writing.

SUE MOSTELLER, C.S.J.

LITERARY EXECUTRIX AND TRUSTEE FOR HENRI NOUWEN LEGACY
TORONTO, ONTARIO

What a precious resource Courage for Caregivers will be for those who give care and compassion. As a family therapist for over 40 years, I have had many occasions to share the works of Henri Nouwen with clients and to see their hearts and minds lifted with hope and strength at times of great pain and distress, and at times of deep joy and fulfillment in the journey of loving another. The guided process for a caregivers retreat is a brilliant and extremely helpful appendix to this beautifully written and illustrated guide for those called to being with, and walking alongside, others.

DIANE MARSHALL, RP, RMFT, *REGISTERED PSYCHOTHERAPIST*

THE INSTITUTE OF FAMILY LIVING, TORONTO

As someone who supports caregivers—those caring for loved ones and those involved in caring professions—I am excited for the opportunity to use this wonderful resource. Courage for Caregivers explores so many of the themes and questions people experience in a caring role. Henri Nouwen's words are treasured gifts that continue to inspire and strengthen, and the stories and reflective format will be invaluable to anyone looking for support in their caregiving roles.

MICHELLE O'ROURKE, RN, *PALLIATIVE CARE NURSE AND EDUCATOR*

AUTHOR OF BEFRIENDING DEATH: HENRI NOUWEN AND A SPIRITUALITY OF DYING

The relationship journeys of caregivers and care receivers are ones we may not or cannot anticipate or plan. We find ourselves in the land of vulnerability and weakness with a need to reorient. One pathway through the unfamiliar is the shared experiences and wisdom of others. Courage for Caregivers does just that. This resource opens up a space for exploration, acceptance, and understanding to find those places of hope, rest, and rediscovery. Through the lens of Henri Nouwen's wisdom, Marjorie J. Thompson shares her own personal journey and draws on the stories of others to reveal both the challenges and the unexpected blessings of hope.

DR. NEIL CUDNEY, DMIN, MTS

DIRECTOR, ORGANIZATIONAL AND SPIRITUAL LIFE, CHRISTIAN HORIZONS
CO-CHAIR, ONTARIO FAITH AND CULTURE INCLUSION NETWORK
PRESIDENT, DIVISION OF RELIGION AND SPIRITUALITY,
AMERICAN ASSOCIATION INTELLECTUAL AND DEVELOPMENTAL DISABILITIES

My true self is rooted in the One who calls me the beloved,
and who says to me, "I love you with an everlasting love."

—HENRI NOUWEN

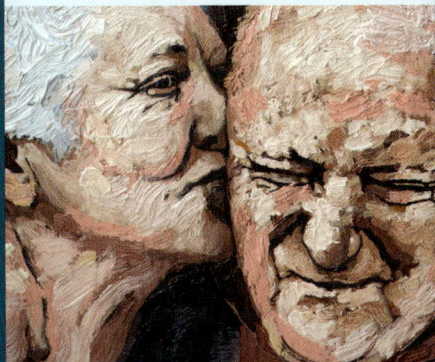

God's deep love is a revitalizing force lifting us when we have no more strength for the challenges of giving care. We see God's love in and through one another.

Share the story of caregiving with your community

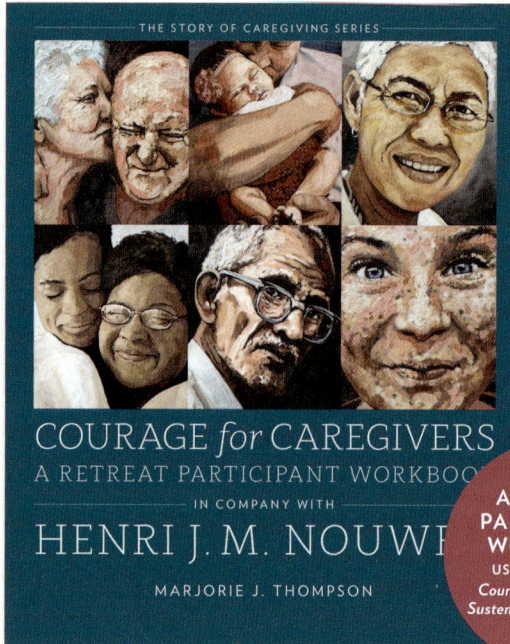

A RETREAT PARTICIPANT WORKBOOK
USED ALONGSIDE
Courage for Caregivers: Sustenance for the Journey

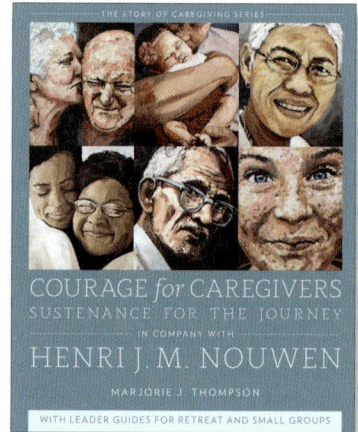

COURAGE FOR CAREGIVERS: SUSTENANCE FOR THE JOURNEY

USED ALONGSIDE THE Retreat Leader Guide (page 91), this inspirational workbook gathers caregivers to a day away to renew the energies and callings of caregiving and reflect on the belovedness they share with the people they care for. With wisdom from Henri Nouwen, *Courage for Caregivers: A Retreat Participant Workbook* invites caregivers to share their stories, and the workbook invites reflection on the gifts of caregiving that bring restoration for the season that lies ahead. At the end of the day, participants take home a workbook to continue journaling the ongoing story into the heart of God and celebrating the love that binds us to one another.

FEATURES

- teaching from the wisdom of Henri Nouwen
- inspirational quotes
- note-taking space
- personal journaling space
- reflection exercises

To order, visit **STORE.CHURCHHEALTH.ORG**

henri nouwen SOCIETY | Church Health